THE
BRIGHT
GIRL
GUIDE

USE YOUR PERIOD TO YOUR ADVANTAGE

BRIGHT GIRL HEALTH
INFORMED. EMPOWERED.

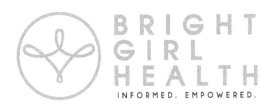

ISBN 978-0-6485853-0-5

Internal graphics by Renee Papadatos

Photography by Sara Eshu

Design by Demi Spaccavento

I vividly remember my first period. It looked absolutely nothing like I'd imagined, in fact, I recall yelling from the bathroom to my mum that she needed to call the doctor - there was something horribly wrong. The 16 page 'puberty' information guide she'd given me some months before did not remotely scratch the surface. As I stared at the mirky (and smelly) mess in my undies, I was left thinking - is this my life now? I felt as if I was living in somebody else's body and I most certainly had no understanding of the intricacies of my menstrual cycle as a 13 year old. It was almost inappropriate to talk about it. All I knew was that a period meant my life was changing, my body was changing but my mind was yet to catch up. I had a lot of learning to do.

I spent most of my teens fearing my body, fertility and my hormones. I had no idea ovulation was the hero of my menses. I was taught that 'being' with a boy at any time would likely end up with an unwanted pregnancy and that period pain was a given. There was very little appreciation for my menstrual cycle because nobody had told or shown me otherwise.

Truth is - I still see this today. Girls are not given the facts because adults fear this knowledge would cause an influx of pregnancies. But I don't think it has always been this way. I'm certain that body wisdom isn't at all new, and women for centuries before us had relied on signs and signals to guide them through their own seasons - from puberty to perimenopause, pregnancy to menopause and beyond. Yet at some point, we disconnected. Be it because of the freedom that birth control offered to us as women or because we got too busy to keep on talking. Something changed. Where we once sat in circles learning and sharing wisdom, we switched it out for moving quickly from one thing to the next, giving little time to what fundamentally shapes us as women. What's interesting is that week after week patients share with me their embarrassment with the little amount of knowledge they have about their cycles, not to mention their disappointment, because they feel robbed for years of unknown vital information that may have lead them towards better health sooner.

As women, whether we like it or not, we are at the mercy of many cycles. Not just the daily motions we go through, but our own rhythmic cycles. We are living within cycles. As seasons pass, our menstrual cycles do too, and each month there is this epically beautiful dance between our hormones, the phases and the stages. Many of us have, at some point, pushed against these cycles. Maybe it's because every month brings pain or maybe your cycles are amiss, or perhaps you bought into the idea that it's an 'inconvenience'. Once we begin to lean in and understand our cycles and our bodies with more curiosity and love, we can pull back the curtain and all of a sudden we see it differently - we can begin to appreciate the gifts it serves to us, like nothing else in this world can offer.

When I finally embraced my own cycle and took my health as my own, life changed for the better. As a Doctor of Chinese Medicine who has seen thousands of women do the same, I have learnt to truly love a woman's body for everything that it is.

I know you want to love and understand your body better - that's why you have invested in this amazing resource. **Demi Spaccavento is such a light in this rapidly growing space of women's health.** I trust that you want this not just for yourself, but for your loved ones and generations to follow. I truly believe that to remove the fear and embrace who we are as women, we need to open up more, ask more questions, but ultimately answer the questions that our children are asking. **I wish I had this information as a young woman** - I wouldn't have had a panic attack on the toilet that day my period arrived or feared the worst for what was to come. **I would have simply understood it was my turn to step into my power as a woman and embrace and celebrate my changing body.** I trust that within these pages lie the clues you need to fully understand and approach your cycle with the love and respect YOU deserve.

Nat Kringoudis
Doctor of Chinese Medicine and
Acupuncture, author, speaker,
founder of The Pagoda Tree clinic.

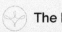

Hi, Bright Girl!

Bright means **intelligent.**
Bright girls are smart. They know their body and they know how to listen to their body.

Bright also means **bold.**
Bright girls are bold and confident. They're not ashamed or scared of their period or their body.

Unfortunately, I know so many girls (and I'm sure you might too) who are embarrassed about their period, especially when they first get it. Think about how many of us hide our pads or tampons when we take them to the bathroom.

NEWS FLASH!
Approximately half the world will experience a period.
On average, women have 450 periods in their lifetime! That is the equivalent of:
448 weeks of periods.
3, 139 days of periods.
70, 080 hours of periods.
8.6 years of periods!

Think back to what you were doing 8.6 years ago.
At the time of writing this, 8.6 years ago I was graduating high school without a clue of what I wanted to do in life. Since then I've studied hard to get my Bachelor and Masters degrees, become a teacher, got married, cut my long hair short and dyed it blonde, and then grew it long again!

8.6 years is a long time.

Considering we spend such a significant amount of our lives on our period, I believe that we need to get better at talking about it and not being ashamed of it.

Those 8.6 years don't have to be spent in misery.
Having a period doesn't have to be a bad experience.
Your period doesn't have to be your enemy.

It is possible to have a symptom free period.
It is possible to improve your hormone health!
YOU CAN HAVE A BETTER PERIOD.

I never want you to feel like you're left in the dark about what is happening with your body.
I want you to have the tools to understand and improve your health.

My hope is that this book will help you have a better period and realise how you can appreciate the amazing and intelligent way your body works.

Demi
Spaccavento

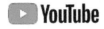
BRIGHT GIRL HEALTH "What is Bright Girl Health?"

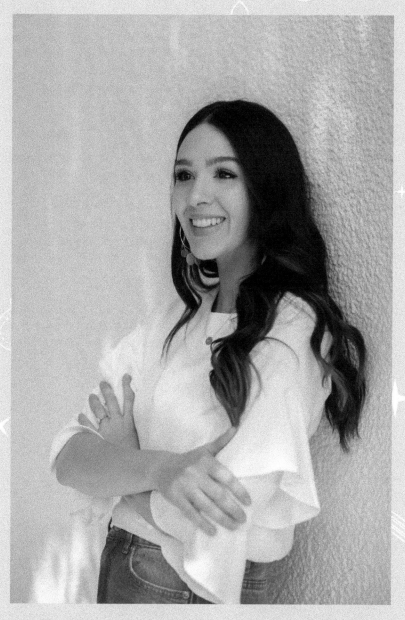

DEMI SPACCAVENTO

is the founder of Bright Girl Health,
a women's health educator,
key note speaker, and a passionate
high school teacher.

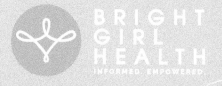

Contents

Reproductive anatomy

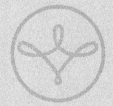

External anatomy

EXTERNAL ANATOMY

Your external reproductive anatomy is what you can see on the outside of the body. Collectively this is referred to as the vulva.

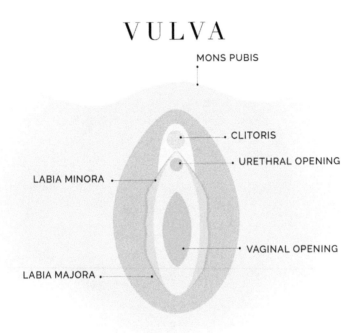

V U L V A

MONS PUBIS

CLITORIS

URETHRAL OPENING

LABIA MINORA

VAGINAL OPENING

LABIA MAJORA

Anatomy	Description
Mons pubis	A mound of fatty tissue beneath pubic hair that protects the internal reproductive organs and is located at the front of the vulva.
Clitoris	A nerve-rich area of the vulva that contributes to sexual sensation.
Urethral opening	The opening from which urine is expelled.
Labia majora	Folds of hair covered skin located below the mons pubis.
Labia minora	Thin, pigmented flaps of skin located in the middle of the labia majora.
Vaginal opening	An opening that leads into the internal reproductive anatomy. The vaginal opening is where menstrual blood is expelled from the body, as well as the opening from which a baby is delivered during labour. This is also the opening in which a penis is inserted during sexual intercourse.

INTERNAL ANATOMY

Your internal reproductive anatomy is inside your body.

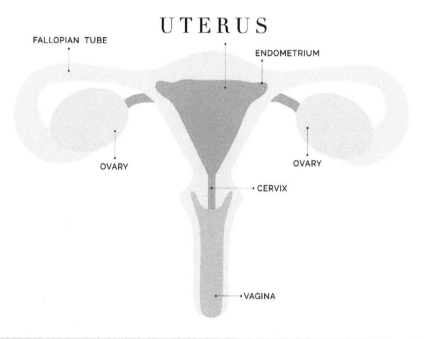

UTERUS

FALLOPIAN TUBE · ENDOMETRIUM · OVARY · OVARY · CERVIX · VAGINA

Anatomy	Description
Vagina/ vaginal canal	A muscular canal (approximately 10cm long) that connects the exterior anatomy to the internal reproductive anatomy. Menstrual blood travels through this canal to exit the body, as does cervical fluid and discharge, and babies during childbirth. This is also where the penis is inserted during intercourse.
Cervix	The 'gateway' to the uterus that projects into the vaginal canal. The cervix produces fluid, which can facilitate the movement of sperm around the female reproductive system.
Uterus	A muscular organ in which a fertilised egg can develop into a fetus.
Fallopian tubes	Ducts through which an ovulated egg will travel to reach the uterus.
Endometrium	The inner lining of the uterus. The innermost layer of the endometrium builds up during the menstrual cycle and then sheds as a period bleed. This process repeats each menstrual cycle.
Ovaries	The female sex organs that house eggs. They also produce hormones such as oestrogen and progesterone.

Your period can reflect a lot about your overall health, and your period symptoms can give you enormous insight into your overall wellbeing

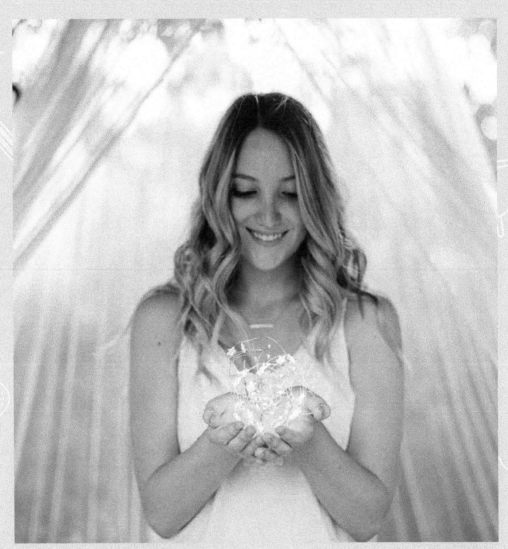

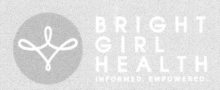

Why a period happens

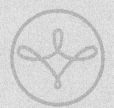

The endometrium

THE ENDOMETRIUM
The endometrium is the innermost layer of the uterus.
It responds to changes in hormones throughout the menstrual cycle. Increasing levels of oestrogen cause the endometrium to build up and thicken. This creates a lining on the uterine walls in which a fertilised egg can potentially implant in order for pregnancy to occur.

The diagram below shows how the endometrium sheds during menstruation, and then slowly thickens throughout the menstrual cycle, until it is shed again at the next period.

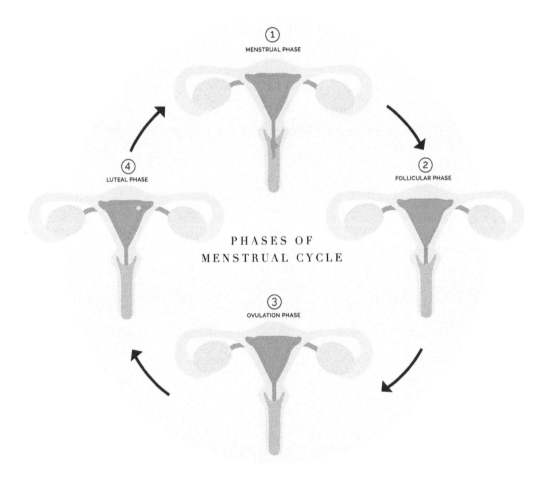

The endometrium

WHY A PERIOD HAPPENS

Most months women do not get pregnant. This means that the uterus does not need the thickened endometrium that was built up throughout the cycle.
The menstrual bleed, or period, is the body expelling the inner layer of the endometrium that it no longer needs. The period bleed is made up of this layer of the endometrium, white blood cells and some mucus.

The diagram below shows the endometrium being shed at the time of menstruation. The period blood exits the body through the vaginal canal.

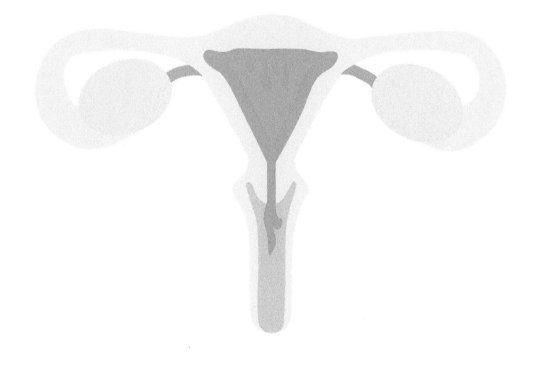

REMEMBER
Your period bleed is the body realising that pregnancy did not occur and it no longer needs the thickened endometrium that was built up, so it is shed.

Making babies

PERIODS AND PREGNANCY

If your menstrual cycle has started your body has the potential to become pregnant, even if you're not sexually active, or you're not ready to be pregnant.
Your eggs have the potential to be released at ovulation time and to be fertilised by a sperm if sexual intercourse takes place.

From the start of your period until the start of the next one, your body is preparing for pregnancy to potentially occur.

Many girls think, "I don't want to get pregnant, so there is no reason to have a period".
While the thought of never having a period again sounds amazing, it is not a good sign for someone to lose their period. As well as allowing pregnancy to be a possibility, your period reflects a lot about your overall health, and your period symptoms can give you enormous insight into your overall wellbeing.

MEET THE FEMALE EGG AND THE MALE SPERM

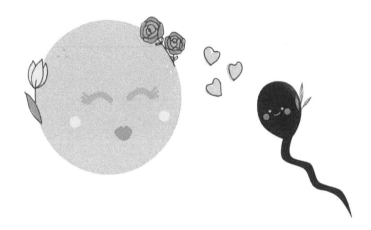

A male sperm can enter the female reproductive system as a result of sexual intercourse. Inside the female reproductive system, sperm have the opportunity to find and unite with an egg if there is one present within the fallopian tubes at the time. This is called fertilisation.

EGG	SPERM
The female reproductive cell containing half the number of chromosomes needed to make a baby	The male reproductive cell containing half the number of chromosomes needed to make a baby

WHAT IS OVULATION?

An egg is released from one of the ovaries each menstrual cycle. Sometimes more than one egg is released, but this is rare. This event is called ovulation.
A woman's ovaries house lots of tiny eggs, which are the female sex cells. Women are born with all the eggs they will ever have. As you get older, thousands of eggs die each year, and some are ovulated. These eggs contain half the number of chromosomes needed to make a baby and are necessary for reproduction.

Once an egg has been released from the ovary, it travels through the fallopian tube and makes its way to the uterus. It is in the fallopian tube that an egg can be fertilised by a male sperm. However, if no sperm is present and fertilisation does not occur, then the egg will degrade within the fallopian tubes or in the uterus after 12-24 hours.

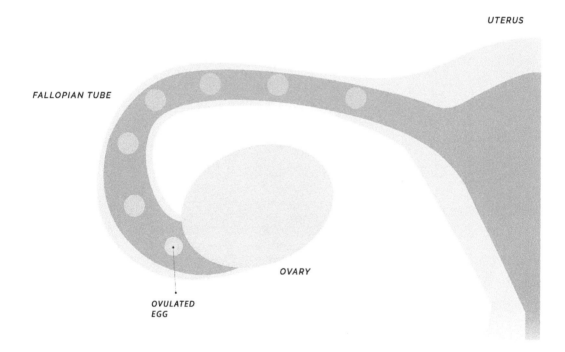

UTERUS

FALLOPIAN TUBE

OVARY

OVULATED
EGG

REMEMBER

Ovulation is when an egg is released from an ovary.
It happens once per menstrual cycle and is needed in order for menstruation (your period) to occur.

Ovulation and the menstrual cycle

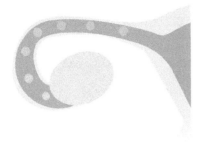

OVULATION NEEDS TO HAPPEN IN ORDER FOR TRUE MENSTRUATION TO HAPPEN

Ovulation has just as much to do with your menstrual cycle as the actual period bleed itself. Ovulation needs to happen in order for a true period to occur.

WHAT IF OVULATION DOESN'T HAPPEN?

A period could go missing if the body fails to ovulate.
Cycles in which ovulation does not take place are called anovulatory cycles. A bleed may sometimes still take place in these cycles, however, this would not be classed as a true menstrual bleed, but is often referred to as an anovulatory bleed.

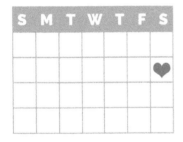

WHEN DOES OVULATION HAPPEN?

Ovulation happens approximately 2 weeks before your next period. This is typically day 14 in the average length cycle, but it will vary from person to person, and even month to month. If someone knows when they are ovulating, they can expect their period approximately 2 weeks later.

THE TIMING OF OVULATION AFFECTS THE TIMING OF YOUR PERIOD

If ovulation happens later, menstruation may happen later.
If ovulation happens earlier, menstruation may happen earlier.

Ovulation in short and long cycles

A TYPICAL LENGTH CYCLE

In the average length menstrual cycle that lasts 28 days, ovulation typically happens around day 14. However, everybody is different, and ovulation doesn't always occur on day 14 for every woman in every cycle.

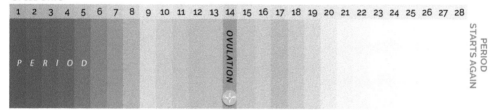

DELAYED OVULATION CYCLE

A period may arrive late if ovulation happens later in a cycle. In this example, ovulation happened on day 20, resulting in a longer than average cycle.

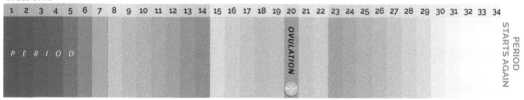

EARLY OVULATION CYCLE

A period may arrive early if ovulation happens earlier in a cycle. In this example, ovulation happened on day 10, resulting in a shorter than average cycle.

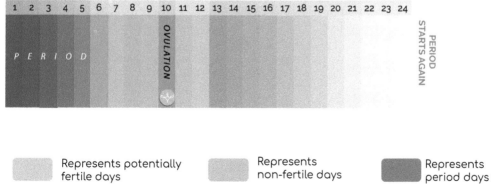

Represents potentially fertile days

Represents non-fertile days

Represents period days

The menstrual cycle

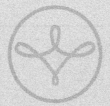

Your period speaks

What might your period say if it could talk?

Maybe it would say...

"Wear the white pants, it will be fine... just kidding!"

or...

"I heard you have a pool party this weekend... it would be a shame if I came and ruined it!"

What about...

"I bled all over your favorite underwear! #sorrynotsorry"

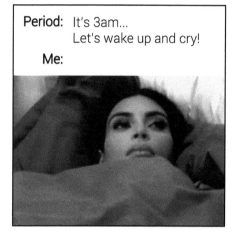

Period: It's 3am...
Let's wake up and cry!

Me:

SIGNS AND SYMPTOMS: YOUR PERIOD'S LANGUAGE

Your body is intelligent and your period can give you *signs and symptoms* that act as an alarm or indicator to let you know an area of your health may need attention.

We might get frustrated at our body when we experience period symptoms like pain, acne, headaches, heavy bleeding or irregular periods. However, it's important that we recognise these symptoms as the body's way of communicating. We should listen to these signs and symptoms instead of getting angry about them.

Signs and symptoms are things you CAN SEE that tell you about things you CANNOT SEE.

WHAT WE CAN SEE (Sign or symptom)	WHAT WE CAN'T SEE (Cause)
Late period	Potentially: Stress, nutrient deficiency, hormone imbalance, etc.
Excess period pain	Potentially: Excess oestrogen, stress, reproductive health condition, etc.

Not just a bleed

The menstrual cycle, is called a cycle for a reason. It includes the *entire cycle* of physical, hormonal and emotional shifts, and changes in the reproductive system. That means the menstrual cycle is not just the days you have a period bleed. At any given time, you are in 1 of 4 phases of this cycle!

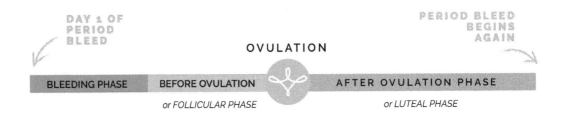

Below is a graph of the hormonal changes that happen in the body throughout the menstrual cycle. Our hormones are constantly moving up and down in relation to one another. Your body and brain use negative feedback loops so that one hormone shifts as a result of changes in other hormones. It is like a beautiful and delicate dance.

HORMONES THROUGHOUT THE MENSTRUAL CYCLE

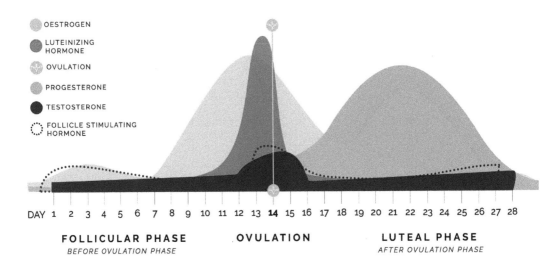

Note: Someone on a hormonal form of contraception like the oral contraceptive pill will not have the same hormone patterns as shown above.

OESTROGEN

Oestrogen is a sex hormone and is produced in larger amounts by females than males. It is predominantly secreted by the ovaries. We have oestrogen receptors in the cells of many parts of our body. Oestrogen is responsible for changes during puberty like breast growth, fat surrounding the hips and stomach, and the growth of pubic hair. It plays an important role in pregnancy and is also an extremely crucial hormone in regulating the menstrual cycle.

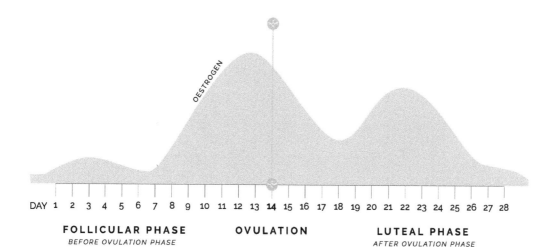

DAY 1 2 3 4 5 6 7 8 9 10 11 12 13 **14** 15 16 17 18 19 20 21 22 23 24 25 26 27 28

FOLLICULAR PHASE
BEFORE OVULATION PHASE

OVULATION

LUTEAL PHASE
AFTER OVULATION PHASE

ROLE OF OESTROGEN IN THE MENSTRUAL CYCLE

- Oestrogen causes the endometrium lining to thicken, which prepares the uterus to receive a fertilised egg so pregnancy can be achieved.
- Oestrogen causes cervical fluid to be produced. When oestrogen levels rise enough the body produces fertile quality cervical fluid (see pages 42-44). This type of cervical fluid makes pregnancy more probable. Low oestrogen levels may see cervical fluid dry up.

- Oestrogen triggers ovulation to happen. Oestrogen levels influence levels of FSH (follicle stimulating hormone) and LH (luteinising hormone). As oestrogen levels rise just prior to ovulation, it triggers the hypothalamus and pituitary gland in the brain to release luteinising hormone. This causes the eggs within the ovaries to mature, leading to ovulation.

Hormones

PROGESTERONE

Progesterone is another sex hormone that is produced in larger amounts by females than males. Progesterone levels are low in the first half of the menstrual cycle, and increase after ovulation. When an egg is released from a follicle on the ovary at ovulation time, the follicle left behind becomes the **corpus luteum**. The corpus luteum is responsible for secreting progesterone in the luteal phase (or 'after ovulation' phase) of the cycle. Progesterone also plays an important role in the establishment and maintenance of pregnancy.

Adequate progesterone levels are important for overall hormone balance. Stress can deplete progesterone levels.

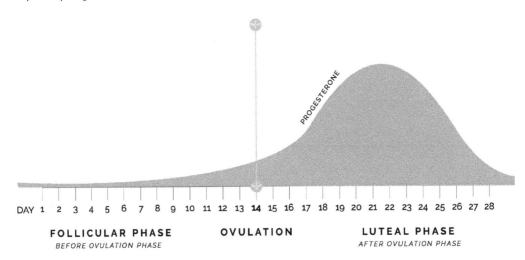

| DAY 1 2 3 4 5 6 7 8 9 10 11 12 13 **14** 15 16 17 18 19 20 21 22 23 24 25 26 27 28 |

FOLLICULAR PHASE
BEFORE OVULATION PHASE

OVULATION

LUTEAL PHASE
AFTER OVULATION PHASE

ROLE OF PROGESTERONE IN THE MENSTRUAL CYCLE

- Progesterone has a balancing effect on oestrogen. Appropriate levels of progesterone in relation to oestrogen are needed for optimal hormone balance.
- Progesterone takes over from oestrogen in the luteal phase and maintains the thickened endometrium so it doesn't shed too early.

- Progesterone can improve fat metabolism and mood.
- Despite PMS symptoms being experienced in the luteal phase where progesterone is highest, unwanted PMS symptoms are not caused by the presence of progesterone. Rather, an imbalance between progesterone and oestrogen may contribute to PMS symptoms.

TESTOSTERONE/ANDROGENS

Testosterone is part of a group of hormones called androgens. Androgens are dominant in males and are responsible for masculinisation. However, they are secreted in women too, but in much smaller amounts. Some androgens are even converted into oestrogen by the body.

Sometimes androgen levels rise higher than what is ideal in females, leading to symptoms like hair growth on the face, acne, defeminisation of body shape and PCOS.

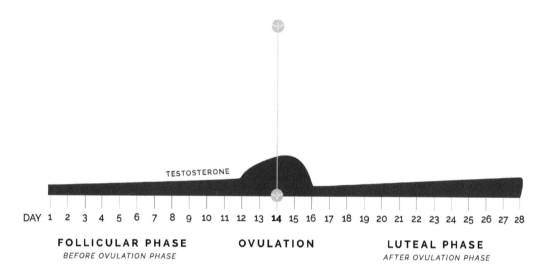

TESTOSTERONE

DAY 1 2 3 4 5 6 7 8 9 10 11 12 13 **14** 15 16 17 18 19 20 21 22 23 24 25 26 27 28

FOLLICULAR PHASE
BEFORE OVULATION PHASE

OVULATION

LUTEAL PHASE
AFTER OVULATION PHASE

ROLE OF ANDROGENS IN THE MENSTRUAL CYCLE

- Androgens are important for growth and development during puberty, therefore, testosterone increases during adolescence.
- Testosterone should remain relatively low throughout the menstrual cycle.

- Testosterone rises around the time of ovulation, which can lead to elevated energy, and increased libido.

FOLLICLE STIMULATING HORMONE

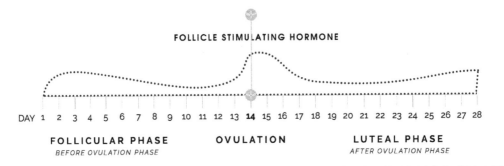

Follicle stimulating hormone (FSH) is released by the pituitary gland in the brain and stimulates the growth of the follicles on the ovaries. These follicles house immature eggs, and FSH helps them to mature and develop in the **follicular** phase of the cycle. Each cycle, one egg matures enough and is ovulated, while others die. FSH production is influenced by oestrogen levels.

LUTEINISING HORMONE

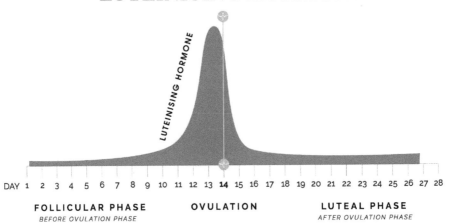

Luteinising hormone (LH) is produced by the pituitary gland in the brain. Rising oestrogen levels send messages to the brain for more LH to be secreted.
When luteinising hormone peaks, it causes ovulation to occur. After ovulation, it decreases because of a rise in progesterone.
The phase in the menstrual cycle after ovulation is also called the **luteal** phase, as luteinising hormone helps the development of the **corpus luteum** (the dying ovarian follicle from which an ovulated egg was released). The corpus luteum is responsible for secreting oestrogen and progesterone in this part of the cycle.

Phases of the menstrual cycle

It's important to know that each phase of the menstrual cycle is very different. You can see on the graph below that the levels of hormones present in our body vary greatly in each of the 4 highlighted sections. Each of these 4 sections represent one of the 4 phases of our menstrual cycle.

The different phases of the menstrual cycle are:

1. The **bleeding phase** OR your period

2. The **follicular phase** OR 'before ovulation' phase

3. The **ovulation phase** - when an ovary releases an egg

4. The **luteal phase** OR 'after ovulation' phase

PHASES THROUGHOUT THE MENSTRUAL CYCLE

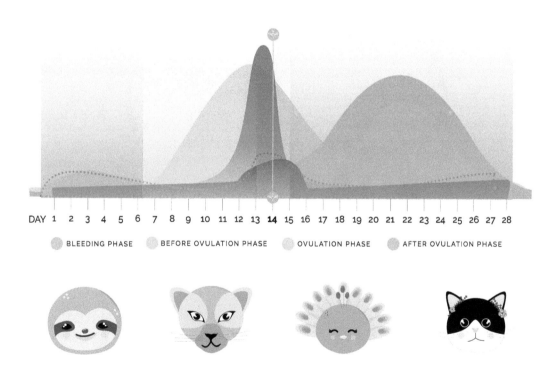

DAY 1 2 3 4 5 6 7 8 9 10 11 12 13 **14** 15 16 17 18 19 20 21 22 23 24 25 26 27 28

BLEEDING PHASE   BEFORE OVULATION PHASE   OVULATION PHASE   AFTER OVULATION PHASE

Phases of the menstrual cycle

These animals help to demonstrate how we might feel in each phase of the menstrual cycle. Considering hormone levels are different in each phase of the cycle, so too will the way we feel **physically, mentally, emotionally, and behaviourally.**
Knowing which phase we're in can help us understand why one week we feel energetic like a lioness, and the next week we might want to stay in bed and sleep 18 hours a day like a cat. When we experience significant changes in how we feel from week to week, it is important to try not to become frustrated with ourselves. Instead, it can improve our relationship with our period to remember what's going on inside our body with our hormones.

We continually move from one phase to the next throughout the cycle, and this process starts again and repeats itself when we get our next period.

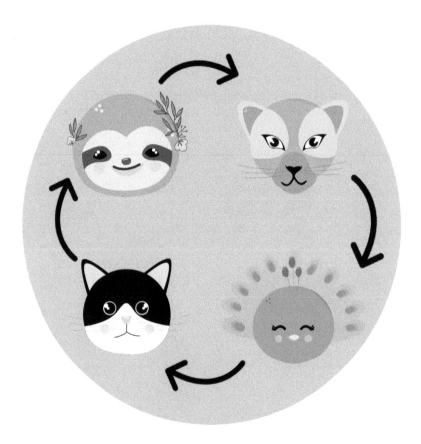

REMEMBER
You may feel different in each phase because of differing hormone levels. WORK WITH IT, NOT AGAINST IT!

Phases of the menstrual cycle

Characteristics of cycle phases

SLOTH PHASE
Menstruation/period bleed

- Includes the days of your period bleed

- Usually lasts 4-7 days

- May feel more tired, slow and inward focussed

- May feel the need for more rest at the beginning of this phase

LIONESS PHASE
Before ovulation

- Starts immediately after your period bleed ends

- Lasts until ovulation time (the length of this phase can vary from person to person)

- May feel more energetic and strong

- May feel more happy and have more stable emotions in this phase

CAT PHASE
After ovulation

- Begins after ovulation has taken place

- Usually lasts 12-16 days. On average, this phase is 14 days leading up to your next period. This phase typically will not vary much in length

- May be characterised by PMS (premenstrual syndrome) symptoms

PEACOCK PHASE
Ovulation

- Roughly 1-3 days surrounding the time an egg is released from an ovary

- Ovulation is typically said to happen around cycle day 14. However, it doesn't always

- Some women may experience ovulation pain, ovulation spotting, or nausea

- May have increases in energy or improved mood

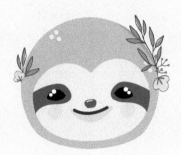

MENSTRUATION
Sloth Phase

WHEN The days of your period bleed

HOW YOU COULD FEEL

- Stomach cramps
- Tiredness
- Food cravings
- Moody or tearful
- Decreased energy
- More withdrawn from social settings
- Decreased performance in sports

SLOTH CHARACTERISTICS

- More inward focussed
- Slower and sleepier
- Need more rest
- Cute and snuggly

WORK WITH IT

- Schedule time for rest
- Exercise appropriately for how your body feels
- Be kind to yourself if you feel emotional
- Know the symptoms to expect

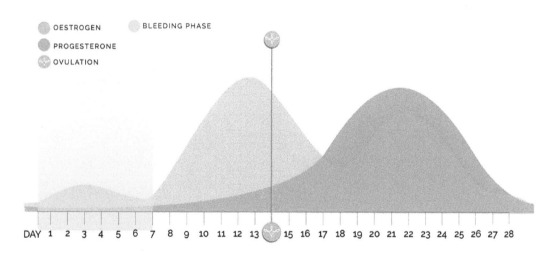

OESTROGEN   BLEEDING PHASE
PROGESTERONE
OVULATION

DAY 1 2 3 4 5 6 7 8 9 10 11 12 13 14 15 16 17 18 19 20 21 22 23 24 25 26 27 28

FOLLICULAR PHASE
BEFORE OVULATION PHASE

OVULATION

LUTEAL PHASE
AFTER OVULATION PHASE

Lower levels of **oestrogen** and **progesterone** trigger the menstrual bleed and cause us to experience period symptoms.

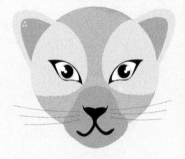

FOLLICULAR
Lioness Phase

LIONESS CHARACTERISTICS
- Strong
- Athletic
- Boss babes - they hunt for the tribe

WHEN   Just after your period stops

HOW YOU COULD FEEL

- More energetic
- Better concentration and brain function
- Minimal cravings
- More social

- More stable emotions & mood
- Heightened athletic performance

WORK WITH IT
- Schedule more social activities
- Get lots of work or assignments done
- Do more sport or exercise

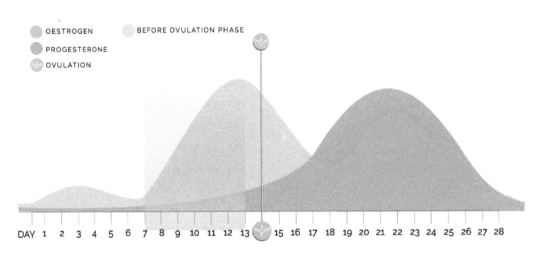

- OESTROGEN
- PROGESTERONE
- OVULATION

BEFORE OVULATION PHASE

DAY 1 2 3 4 5 6 7 8 9 10 11 12 13 14 15 16 17 18 19 20 21 22 23 24 25 26 27 28

FOLLICULAR PHASE
BEFORE OVULATION PHASE

OVULATION

LUTEAL PHASE
AFTER OVULATION PHASE

Rising levels of **testosterone** and **oestrogen** can make us feel more energetic in this phase.

OVULATION
Peacock Phase

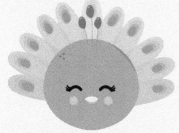

PEACOCK CHARACTERISTICS
- Beautiful
- Flirty

Peacocks spread their feathers to attract a mate. For humans, the ovulation phase is the time when mating can result in pregnancy.

WHEN During ovulation.
This phase only lasts around 1-3 days

HOW YOU COULD FEEL

- More energetic
- Better concentration and brain function
- Minimal cravings
- More social
- Some women experience ovulation pain or spotting (small amount of bleeding)

WORK WITH IT
- Look for ovulation signs and track them
- Schedule more social activities
- Get lots of work or study done
- Do more sport or exercise

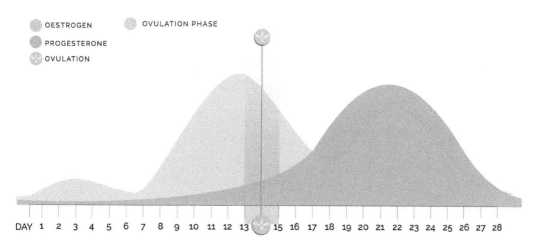

- OESTROGEN
- PROGESTERONE
- OVULATION
- OVULATION PHASE

DAY 1 2 3 4 5 6 7 8 9 10 11 12 13 14 15 16 17 18 19 20 21 22 23 24 25 26 27 28

FOLLICULAR PHASE
BEFORE OVULATION PHASE

OVULATION

LUTEAL PHASE
AFTER OVULATION PHASE

High levels of **testosterone** and **oestrogen** can make us feel more energetic in this phase.

The 'after ovulation' (luteal) phase

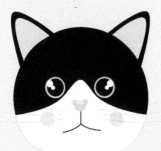

LUTEAL
Cat Phase

WHEN After ovulation has occurred
Approximately 2 weeks leading up to period

HOW YOU COULD FEEL

- PMS symptoms
- Decreased energy
- Decreased concentration & brain function
- Breast swelling or pain
- Tiredness
- Mood swings
- Crying
- Headaches
- Feelings of anxiety/depression

CAT CHARACTERISTICS
- Cuddly one minute, cold the next
- Rest & sleep often

WORK WITH IT
- Schedule time for rest
- Be kind to yourself when you feel emotional
- Adjust exercise according to how you feel

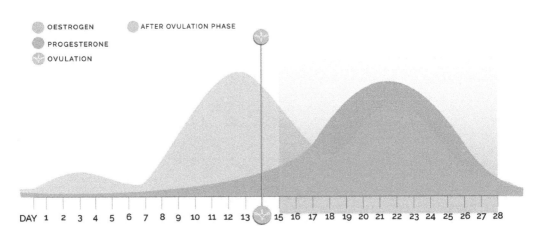

- OESTROGEN
- PROGESTERONE
- OVULATION
- AFTER OVULATION PHASE

DAY 1 2 3 4 5 6 7 8 9 10 11 12 13 14 15 16 17 18 19 20 21 22 23 24 25 26 27 28

FOLLICULAR PHASE
BEFORE OVULATION PHASE

OVULATION

LUTEAL PHASE
AFTER OVULATION PHASE

Progesterone takes over from oestrogen in this part of the cycle. This hormone shift can contribute to PMS symptoms.

Tracking your menstrual cycle

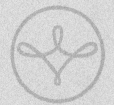

Knowing which phase you're in

HOW TO KNOW WHICH PHASE YOU'RE IN

It's easy to know when you're in your bleeding (sloth) phase... you're literally bleeding and that's pretty hard to miss!

After your period stops, you immediately enter the before ovulation (lioness) phase. But how do you know when the ovulation (peacock) phase starts and when you transition into the after ovulation (cat) phase?

By reading your period signs and symptoms!

TRACKING PERIOD SIGNS AND SYMPTOMS

I believe every girl should be tracking her menstrual cycle.

Tracking the characteristics of each of the 4 cycle phases, and any additional signs or symptoms, will help you to identify which phase of your cycle you are in.

Ovulation tracking can also be used to determine when you're in the ovulation (peacock) phase, and when your 'after ovulation' (cat) phase begins.

Contrary to what a lot of women practise, tracking your period doesn't just mean writing down when your period bleed starts and when it ends.

It is more effective to track your *entire cycle* throughout all four phases. This is literally all the time because you are always in 1 of the 4 phases of the menstrual cycle. It could seem like a lot of effort to keep track of your signs and symptoms every day. However, it only takes a few minutes to enter your observations into an app or onto a paper chart. You can do this on the toilet, while brushing your teeth or as part of your bedtime routine.

3 REASONS TO TRACK YOUR CYCLE

It will help to more accurately predict when to expect your next period

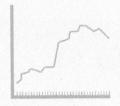

It will potentially help a health professional diagnose any irregularities more accurately if you were to show them your chart

It helps you feel more in tune with your body and your emotions

Tracking in an app

APPS TO TRACK YOUR PERIOD

There are many apps, both free and paid, that you can use to track your menstrual cycle. You can keep track of any patterns that may form by recording any signs and symptoms you observe in the apps. These patterns can give you and a health professional valuable insight into your hormonal health and how you might be able to improve your hormone balance and have a better period.

These apps below are great options for period tracking because they give a graph overview of your data at the end of the month. This helps you to visually identify any patterns that emerge.

Note: Some period tracking apps will try to predict when you will ovulate. These predictions are not always accurate. A more reliable way of tracking ovulation is to use the strategies in the next chapter. However, apps are still a useful tool for keeping track of your period signs/symptoms.

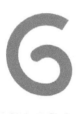

GLOW

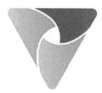

KINDARA

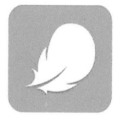

FLO

PERIOD SIGNS AND SYMPTOMS TO TRACK:

- When your period starts/finishes
- If your period is heavy or light
- Moods and mood swings
- Colour and consistency of menstrual blood
- Food cravings and appetite
- Bloating and digestion symptoms
- Concentration levels
- Anxiety symptoms
- Energy levels

- Pelvic pain/upper leg pain/back pain
- Acne breakouts
- Headaches
- Sore/swollen breasts
- Diarrhea or constipation
- Sleep patterns
- Basal body temperature
- Cervical fluid changes

Tracking

ovulation

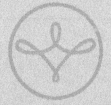

Why track ovulation?

The body will give observable signs to communicate that you are ovulating. The female body is very intelligent.

Many of us are not taught about how to watch for these signs, and we end up missing them. This is such a shame because when we know how to listen to our body and know how to interpret the 'language' it speaks, then we can use our period to our advantage! For example, we can schedule important events around the time of ovulation, as this is the time we typically feel best. Recognising ovulation signs can also save you from the confusion or stress you may feel when you see differences in the cervical fluid that can be observed in your underwear throughout your cycle.

3 REASONS TO TRACK OVULATION

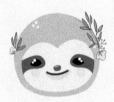

KNOW WHICH PHASE YOU'RE IN
Tracking ovulation helps you clearly identify which phase of your cycle you're in. Knowing ovulation is happening helps determine when you will enter your 'after ovulation' phase.

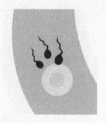

PREGNANCY ACHIEVEMENT OR PREVENTION
If trained to properly track ovulation, women can use this knowledge to support pregnancy achievement or pregnancy prevention. The time surrounding ovulation is the window in which pregnancy can occur. Timing intercourse to coincide with ovulation increases the chance of pregnancy.

PREDICT WHEN EVEN THE MOST IRREGULAR PERIODS WILL ARRIVE
Even if your period is irregular, ovulation will typically happen approximately 14 days before your next period (with a few exceptions). Whether your cycle is 28 days long, 21 days long, or 80 days long, if you know when ovulation happens, you can expect to get your period 2 weeks later.

When you know how to listen to your body and know how to interpret the 'language' it speaks...

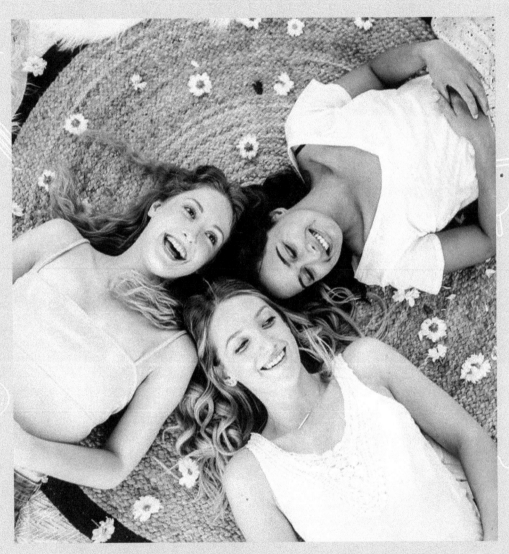

... then you can use your period to your advantage!

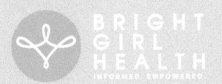

BRIGHT GIRL HEALTH
INFORMED. EMPOWERED.

Basal body temperature

After ovulation occurs and an egg has been released from one of the ovaries, the follicle from which it was released starts to produce the hormone **progesterone**. Progesterone produces heat.
This means that after ovulation has taken place, body temperature will increase because of the increasing amount of progesterone being produced.

This increase in temperature is referred to as a **temperature shift** and can be observed by recording your basal body temperature daily.

> **Basal Body Temperature**
> The lowest body temperature attained during rest. It is taken after waking from a full night's sleep, before any form of physical activity, eg: walking to the bathroom.

Basal body temperature (BBT) should be recorded first thing in the morning immediately after waking up and before exerting much physical energy. Even getting up to go to the bathroom before taking your temperature could potentially alter the reading. Some women are more sensitive to their BBT readings being impacted by factors like moving around, or variations to the time at which temperature is taken.
You can use most thermometers that record to 2 decimal places (Celsius) or 1 decimal place (Fahrenheit) to track your BBT orally. There are also thermometers you can purchase that are designed specifically for ovulation tracking.

This is an example of a BBT chart with a clear temperature increase after ovulation occurs.

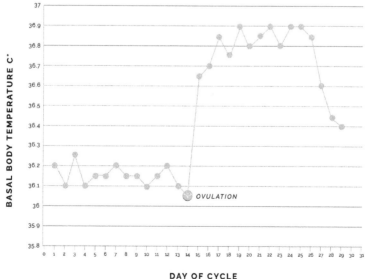

DAY OF CYCLE

Basal body temperature

OBSERVING A TEMPERATURE SHIFT

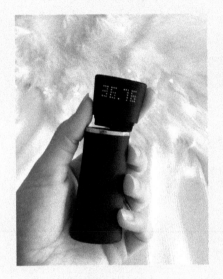

1. Record body temperature to **2 decimal places Celsius or 1 decimal place Farenheit** at approximately the same time each morning immediately after waking up.

2. Record your daily temperature reading on a paper chart or in a dedicated period tracking app.

3. Watch for a temperature shift. This will be an increase in temperature of 0.11 degrees (C) or 0.2 degrees (F) above the previous day's temperature.
   To count as a temperature shift it should also be 0.05 degrees (C) or 0.1 degrees (F) higher than the temperature recordings from the 6 days prior.

4. Continue watching your temperatures for the next **3 days** to ensure they remain higher than the temperatures prior to the shift.

REMEMBER

Basal body temperature should rise the day after ovulation. This is called a temperature shift.

The last day of low temperatures is likely the day on which ovulation took place.

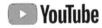 **BRIGHT GIRL HEALTH** "Basal body temperature to track your period cycle"

Basal body temperature

The graphs below show that just like progesterone rises after ovulation, so does basal body temperature.

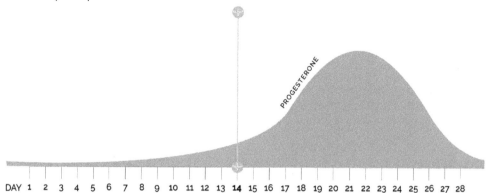

BBT CHART

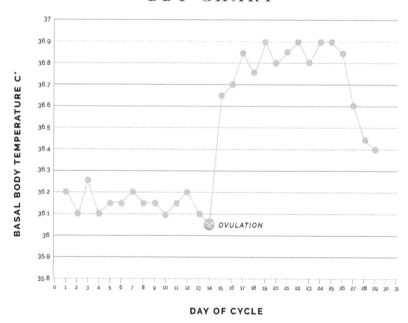

DAY OF CYCLE

The temperatures on this chart are under 36.27 degrees Celsius before ovulation. Ovulation happened on day 14. The rise in progesterone after ovulation caused basal body temperature to rise at least 0.11 degrees (C). The next 3 postovulatory temperatures remain at least 0.05 degrees (C) higher than the 6 temperatures prior to ovulation. These factors confirm that ovulation took place.

This is not intended as official training in BBT tracking.

CERVICAL FLUID

Cervical fluid is mucus secreted by your cervix that changes in consistency and colour in response to hormone changes throughout the menstrual cycle.
It is often referred to as discharge, however, cervical fluid is a more appropriate name, as "discharge" can refer to a number of different types of vaginal secretions that are not necessarily cervical fluid.

Cervical fluid can be seen in underwear or on toilet paper after wiping. *Cervical fluid is normal* and can be a helpful way that the body communicates about what is going on with the health of your vagina, cervix and hormones.

THE ROLE OF CERVICAL FLUID

The role that cervical fluid plays will change throughout menstrual cycle.
If we simplify it, cervical fluid has 2 roles:
1. At certain times in the menstrual cycle cervical fluid helps sperm live and move within the female reproductive system
2. At other times, cervical fluid makes the vaginal environment inhospitable to sperm or causes them to die more quickly

TYPES OF CERVICAL FLUID

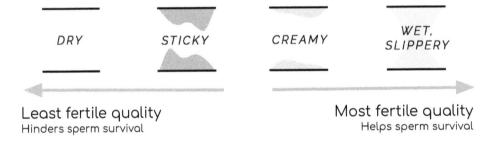

DRY STICKY CREAMY WET, SLIPPERY

Least fertile quality
Hinders sperm survival

Most fertile quality
Helps sperm survival

UNHEALTHY DISCHARGE

While cervical fluid is a healthy sign of the menstrual cycle, sometimes women can notice discharge that is indicative of an infection. This is NOT cervical fluid.
Discharge that could indicate infection:

- May have a tint of colour (yellowish, greenish)
- May be foul smelling
- May be an abnormal consistency (perhaps lumpy or like cottage cheese)
- May be accompanied by symptoms such as burning, itching or pain

If you observe any of these signs or experience these symptoms, you should see your doctor and check for infection.

Cervical fluid

CHANGES IN CERVICAL FLUID AT OVULATION TIME

Changes in cervical fluid can help to determine where you are in your menstrual cycle.

As ovulation approaches, cervical fluid starts to change.

For the majority of the month cervical fluid works to keep sperm away from the uterus by making the vaginal environment inhabitable. However, in the days leading up to ovulation, oestrogen levels rise. The body responds to this rise in oestrogen and starts to make fertile quality cervical fluid. This is the kind of cervical fluid that keeps sperm alive.

As ovulation approaches, the opportunity for a sperm to find an egg and fertilise it is drawing near, and the body intelligently starts to create an environment within the vagina that will allow sperm to survive.

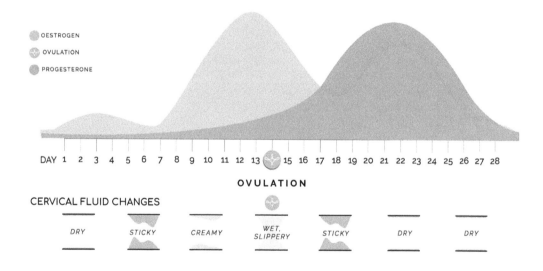

● OESTROGEN
● OVULATION
● PROGESTERONE

DAY 1 2 3 4 5 6 7 8 9 10 11 12 13 ● 15 16 17 18 19 20 21 22 23 24 25 26 27 28

OVULATION

CERVICAL FLUID CHANGES

| DRY | STICKY | CREAMY | WET. SLIPPERY | STICKY | DRY | DRY |

Example: Cervical fluid is mostly dry when the body is not fertile. As ovulation draws near and the body is approaching it's most fertile time of the month, cervical fluid changes to gradually become more wet and resemble a sticky, creamy or wet/slippery consistency.
This is reflected on the graph above.

Note: Each woman's cervical fluid consistency and patterns may look different. Some women may also see wetter cervical fluid in the lead up to a period due to a progesterone peak. Some may see cervical fluid all month round and some may struggle to observe cervical fluid because they produce very little.

Cervical fluid

FERTILE QUALITY CERVICAL FLUID

Fertile quality cervical fluid is the type of cervical fluid that allows for sperm survival inside the female reproductive system. The presence of fertile quality cervical fluid increases fertility and the chance of pregnancy occurring.

WET,
SLIPPERY

Fertile quality cervical fluid is produced as ovulation approaches and is:
- Stretchy - can be stretched between 2 fingers without easily breaking
- Wet and slippery
- Can look like raw egg white

This type of cervical fluid is commonly referred to as 'egg white' cervical fluid, because it closely resembles the look and feel of raw egg white.

INTERPRET WHAT CERVICAL FLUID MEANS

- Observe cervical fluid by looking in your underwear or on toilet paper after wiping. Some women may use their fingers to find cervical fluid, but this is not necessary. You can also use sensation/feel to reinforce cervical fluid observations as wet/slippery/egg white fluid may also make you feel more wet.
- When you observe fertile quality cervical fluid, it indicates that your body is getting ready to ovulate or it is ovulating.
- On the day after you ovulate, fertile quality cervical fluid will disappear, or decrease in fertile quality, indicating that ovulation has taken place.

The exception to this rule is if you notice fertile quality cervical fluid and then it goes away, only to return again a few days later. This can indicate an attempt at ovulation that was not successful. Fertile quality cervical fluid reappearing can mean that your body is making another attempt at ovulation.
Observing basal body temperature changes in conjunction with cervical fluid can help you to determine if ovulation has successfully taken place or not. A temperature shift will indicate successful ovulation.

Remember, *everybody is different!*
Some women may not see cervical fluid that resembles egg white, or may not produce as much as others. It is important for every woman to get to know her body's own pattern of cervical fluid with observation and practice.

Ovulation signs

READ THE SIGNS

Now that you know how your body can communicate when ovulation is happening, you can use it to your advantage!

It feels empowering to be able to understand when your own body is telling you that it is ovulating. This is one of a woman's greatest super powers!

If you can listen to your body in this way, then you can better predict when your next period will be and never be caught unprepared! You may even be able to notice if your body does not ovulate one month, or if ovulation comes unusually late or early. This can help you identify any health concerns early on, to help you maintain your health throughout your life.

Below is a summary of the signs to look out for to determine when ovulation is happening:

BASAL BODY TEMPERATURE	CERVICAL FLUID CHANGES	OTHER FERTILITY SIGNS
A shift (increase) in basal body temperature will indicate that ovulation has successfully taken place.	Cervical fluid becoming more wet in consistency will indicate that ovulation is coming.	• Cervical position • Ovulation pain • Ovulation spotting • Increased energy • Swollen vaginal lips • Breast tenderness
Your body temperature will rise the day after you ovulate.	'Egg white' or wet cervical fluid can indicate that the body is getting ready to ovulate or is ovulating.	And more! You may experience some of the above, or none of them. Everyone is different!
The last day of low temperatures is likely the day on which ovulation took place.	Cervical fluid will decrease in fertile quality for the rest of the cycle after ovulation has taken place.	

Fertility and pregnancy

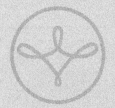

How pregnancy happens

PREGNANCY CAN'T HAPPEN WITHOUT OVULATION

For an egg to be fertilised by a sperm and for pregnancy to occur, ovulation needs to take place.

An ovulated egg is released from an ovary where it cannot be fertilised. It travels through the fallopian tube where it can potentially be fertilised by a sperm.

No ovulation = No egg

No egg = No pregnancy

The days around ovulation is the window of time that the female body is most fertile. This is when pregnancy is most likely to occur.

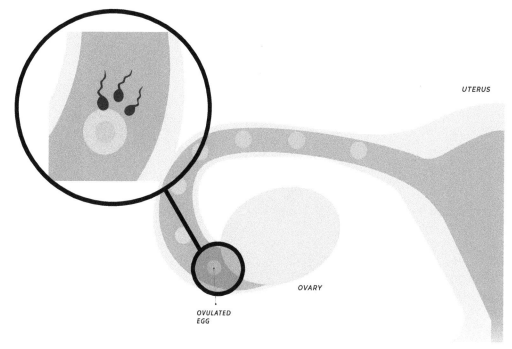

UTERUS

OVARY

OVULATED
EGG

Sperm make their way through the female reproductive system in search of an ovulated egg. Only one sperm will be able to fertilise an egg.

REMEMBER

AN EGG LIVES FOR ONLY AROUND 12-24 HOURS AFTER OVULATION.

This is the time in which a sperm has the opportunity to find and fertilise an egg for pregnancy to be achieved. If fertilisation does not occur, the opportunity is missed until the next ovulation phase.

How pregnancy happens

HOW PREGNANCY HAPPENS

When a sperm from a male meets an ovulated egg from a female, they unite to form a zygote. This happens as a result of sexual intercourse.

The zygote must now implant into the lining of the uterus (endometrium) in order for pregnancy to be achieved.

There is a high occurrence of fertilised eggs failing to implant, in which case, pregnancy does not occur and the egg is shed with the next period bleed.

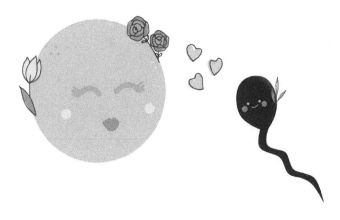

TERMS	DESCRIPTION
Egg and sperm	<u>Gamete</u> - Contains half the number of chromosomes needed to form a zygote.
Fertilised egg	<u>Zygote</u> - The egg and sperm fuse and form a fertilised egg containing all the genetic material needed for a baby.
Pregnancy	An egg has been fertilised, has successfully implanted into the wall of the uterus and is developing into a baby.

Note: Pregnancy happens as a result of sexual intercouse when the penis is inserted into the vagina. Oral sex and other sexual acts do not allow for pregnancy to occur.

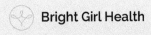

Fertilisation and implantation

PREGNANCY ACHIEVEMENT

Pregnancy is achieved in 2 steps:

1. *Fertilisation* - a sperm and an egg unite.
2. *Implantation* - a fertilised egg has successfully implanted in the uterus and is developing into a baby.

IT'S SIMPLE MATH...

Egg + Sperm = Zygote (fertilised egg)

Zygote + implantation in uterus = Pregnancy

FERTILISATION AND IMPLANTATION

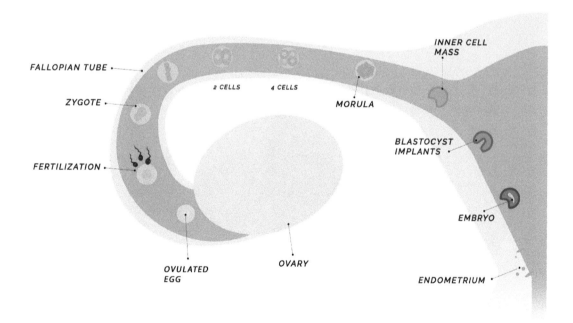

The female reproductive system is constantly going about the work of fertility.

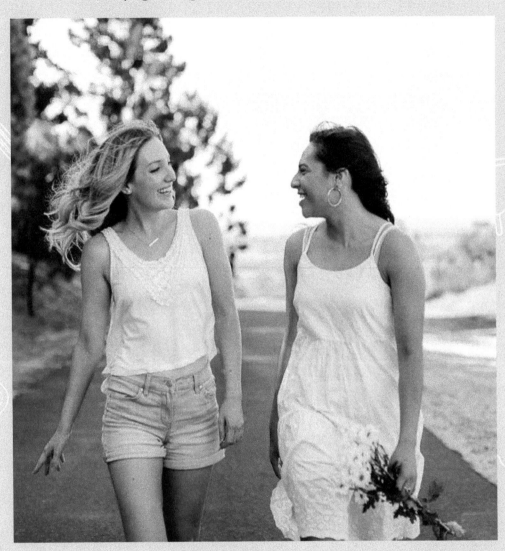

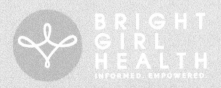

What is fertility?

FERTILITY

Put simply, fertility is someone's ability to conceive and produce offspring. In other words, it's someone's potential to get pregnant.
As my friend Nat Kringoudis says, *"fertility isn't just about babies"*.
Whether you want to become pregnant right now or not, your fertility is a bigger part of your overall health than you may think!

Your health affects your fertility and your fertility can be reflective of your health.
A healthy period can also be a sign of good fertility.

Interestingly, women are not fertile (able to become pregnant) all month round.

THE DIFFERENCE BETWEEN GUYS & GIRLS

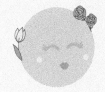 Females produce
1
egg per menstrual
cycle

 Males produce
200
million
sperm per day

FERTILITY THROUGHOUT THE MENSTRUAL CYCLE

Females release 1 egg from an ovary only once per menstrual cycle (with the less common exception of more than 1 egg being released at ovulation time, which is not the usual).
When an egg is released at ovulation, this is the small window of time in which it can be fertilised by a sperm for pregnancy to occur. After ovulation, an egg will typically survive for a period of 12-24 hours, after which it will break down, and the chance for pregnancy has passed until ovulation time in the next cycle.

Just because women only ovulate once per cycle does not mean that they are 'infertile' the rest of their cycle.
Throughout the entire menstrual cycle the body works towards ovulation, builds up the endometrium to potentially receive a fertilised egg, and prepares for a potential pregnancy to occur.
The female reproductive system is constantly going about the work of fertility.

When can pregnancy occur?

FEMALE FERTILE PHASE

The days in the menstrual cycle on which sexual intercourse (or even insemination) could result in pregnancy are referred to as the **female fertile phase,** or even the **fertile window.**

Pregnancy cannot occur on every day of a woman's menstrual cycle. The days on which pregnancy can occur revolve around ovulation time and account for the lifespan of the female egg and male sperm.

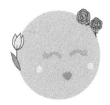

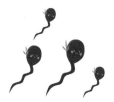

An egg lives for
12-24 HOURS
After ovulation

Sperm live up to
5 DAYS
Inside the female body after intercourse

WHEN ARE WE FERTILE?

The female fertile window is roughly the 5 days before ovulation, and the 2-3 days after ovulation.

- **5 days before ovulation** - This takes into account the potential for sperm to live inside the female reproductive system for up to 5 days in the right conditions, especially when there is fertile quality cervical fluid present.

- **2-3 days after ovulation** - This takes into account the lifespan of an ovulated egg of up to 24 hours. The 2nd and 3rd day also account for the possibility of a second egg being released at ovulation time (not too common, but possible) or the possibility that the day of ovulation was incorrectly identified.

Pregnancy: Not as easy as it seems

When someone isn't ready to become pregnant, it can seem like pregnancy can happen easily.

However, as we can see from this 'Fertile phase within the menstrual cycle' timeline, there are actually more days in the average menstrual cycle where a woman is NOT fertile, than there are where she IS fertile.

In this timeline, the pink days represent fertile days, the grey days are non-fertile days, and the red days are period bleed days.

Fertile phase within the menstrual cycle

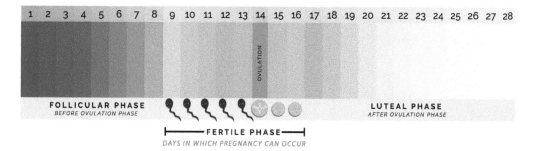

The pink days on the timeline above represent the days on which this person, who ovulated on day 14 of her cycle, is potentially fertile or able to become pregnant as a result of intercourse. The 3rd day after ovulation is sometimes also considered potentially fertile.

Note: The possibility of conception is also impacted by the presence of fertile quality cervical fluid. The case of spontaneous ovulation should also be considered when determining fertility. It is important to remember that not everybody ovulates on day 14. This is an example timeline. Not every cycle will look the same.

INFERTILITY

Infertility in women refers to the inability to conceive or maintain a pregnancy. Some women encounter more obstacles in achieving pregnancy, as there are many factors that need to align to create fertility; regular ovulation, building a thick endometrium ready for implantation, producing cervical fluid to allow for sperm survival, age, overall health, maintaining a pregnancy once conception has occurred... and we haven't even mentioned the fertility of a male partner yet. Contrary to what a lot of people believe, it's not always easy for pregnancy to occur. The good news is that there is always something that can be done to improve fertility. The first step is connecting with a health professional (more on that on pages 72-74).

Getting pregnant on your period

CAN SOMEONE GET PREGNANT WHILE THEY HAVE THEIR PERIOD?

Although becoming pregnant as a result of having intercourse during a woman's menstrual bleed is not common, it is possible.

Women who have a shorter than average menstrual cycle (eg: a 24 day cycle or shorter) have an increased chance of becoming pregnant as a result of sexual intercourse during their period. This is because their fertile phase overlaps with their bleeding days, as shown in the timeline below. In this example, if sexual intercourse takes place on **day 5, 6 or 7,** which are both period days and fertile days, there is an increased potential for pregnancy to occur.

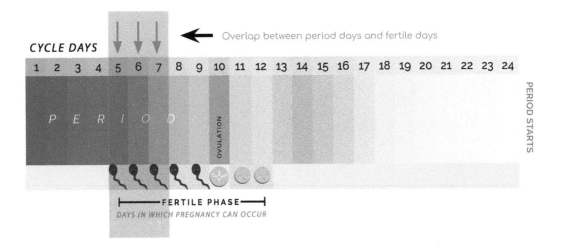

In an average length cycle (28 days), the fertile phase usually starts shortly after bleeding stops and they do not overlap.

Someone with a longer than average menstrual cycle (>28-29 days) isn't likely to become pregnant as a result of intercourse during their period, as their bleeding days and fertile phase don't overlap, as seen in the example below.

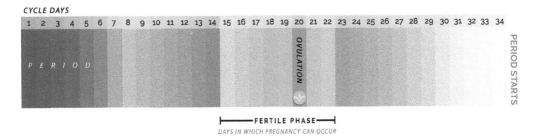

Note: Women may experience a bleed that they interpret to be menstruation that is in fact not menstruation (eg: ovulation spotting or irregular bleeding). This can cause a misinterpretation of when their bleeding phase or their fertile phase actually is. If someone is trying to achieve or avoid pregnancy by tracking their fertile phase they should do so alongside, or after training with, a professional.

Period irregularities

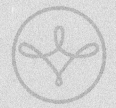

Period irregularities

WHAT ARE PERIOD IRREGULARITIES?

A period irregularity is when a menstrual cycle includes characteristics that are significantly different from that of a typical cycle. Period irregularities usually present as unwanted symptoms that make having a period more frustrating or inconvenient. They can negatively impact your life, studies, relationships, mental health and overall health... and they're annoying!

Most women will probably experience period irregularities in their lifetime. Irregular periods are more expected during teenage years, up until age 18. This is because the body is still getting used to making a period happen regularly with minimal symptoms.

Experiencing occasional irregularities is not always a cause for concern. However, persisting irregularities that are painful or frustrating can be indicative of an underlying health issue that needs to be addressed.

Irregularities are your body's way of communicating something about your health. This is why it is important to monitor any period irregularities by charting them, looking for patterns that may arise, and sharing this information with a professional. By investigating the *cause* of irregularities, you can uncover the reason they arise in the first place and work to have a better period by supporting your body and giving it what it needs.

Common period irregularities

- PMS symptoms
- Period pain
- Acne
- Heavy periods OR light periods
- Missing periods
- Infrequent periods
- Migraines or fainting

BUT DON'T GET MAD AT YOUR BODY!

These irregularities are SYMPTOMS of an underlying cause.
They are not the root problem itself.
It is important to find the root cause of these symptoms.

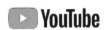 BRIGHT GIRL HEALTH "To my teenage self (advice about periods)"

Hormone imbalance

Why might hormones be out of balance?

- Stress
- Nutrient deficiency – poor diet or poor nutrient absorption
- Overall poor health or gut health
- Eating disorders
- Existing health conditions
- Genetics
- Excess exercise or training at a high level (common amongst teens)
- Environmental oestrogens

Most period irregularities arise because of a hormone imbalance. There could be many reasons why hormones might be out of balance, and these reasons need to be uncovered. When speaking to a health practitioner, ask them to help you investigate the root causes of your period symptoms.

Hormone balance is like a delicate and beautiful dance. As one hormone goes up, another goes down. When certain hormones get high enough, they will trigger the body to release other hormones. When some hormones fall low enough, it will signal to the body to stop producing other hormones.
Our health, stress levels, the environment, and other factors can throw off this delicate balance and lead to hormone imbalance.

Here are some of the main hormones that control the menstrual cycle and the patterns they take in a typical cycle.

HORMONES THROUGHOUT THE MENSTRUAL CYCLE

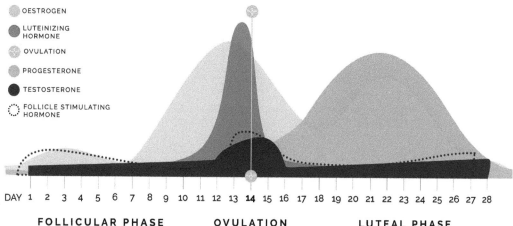

- OESTROGEN
- LUTEINIZING HORMONE
- OVULATION
- PROGESTERONE
- TESTOSTERONE
- FOLLICLE STIMULATING HORMONE

DAY 1 2 3 4 5 6 7 8 9 10 11 12 13 **14** 15 16 17 18 19 20 21 22 23 24 25 26 27 28

FOLLICULAR PHASE
BEFORE OVULATION PHASE

OVULATION

LUTEAL PHASE
AFTER OVULATION PHASE

Hormone balance is like a delicate and beautiful dance

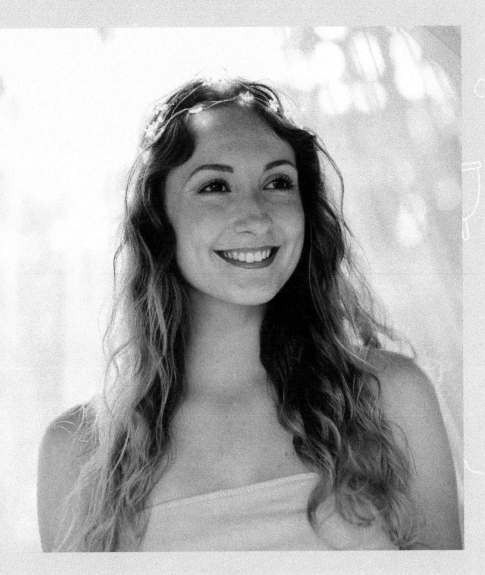

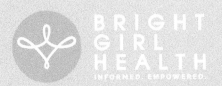

The HPO axis refers to the communication between:

- The <u>H</u>ypothalamus - found in the brain and releases hormones

- The <u>P</u>ituitary gland - found directly under the hypothalamus and also releases hormones

- The <u>O</u>varies - found in the female internal reproductive system and produce sex hormones

The H, P and Os are the dream team that's in charge of making a period happen regularly, on time, and with minimal symptoms. The hormones from the hypothalamus talk to the pituitary gland, and the pituitary gland tells the ovaries to produce hormones, such as oestrogen, which control your period.

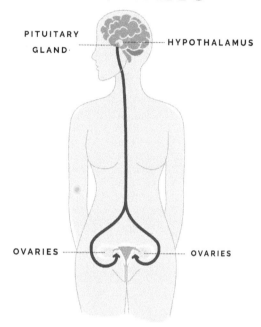

Up until a girl gets her first period, the hypothalamus, pituitary gland and ovaries have never needed to communicate with each other to make a period happen. When a girl gets her first period all of a sudden the H, P and Os have a new job to do together that they've never done before. While someone is still in the first few years of having a period, their HPO axis is described as immature. This is why period irregularities can be more common amongst teenagers. It may take a while for the body to get the hang of having a regular period. In fact, it can take up to 6 years because your hormones have a new job they are still learning.

With time the HPO axis matures and irregular periods in teenagers should improve, providing there are no other health issues preventing this.
Aim for balanced hormones over time, and monitor any irregularities at present.

THE GOOD NEWS - IT GETS BETTER!
Immature HPO axis = More period irregularities
Mature HPO axis = Less period irregularities

Period pain

Statistics reflect that up to **80%** of women experience period pain, varying from mild to disabling pain. It is one of the most common period frustrations women experience. However, just because it's common, doesn't mean that it should be accepted as normal.

Period pain should definitely not interfere with completing everyday tasks, and it should not stop you from living your life the way you want.

TREATING PERIOD PAIN

There is always something that can be done to treat pain and improve your experience of having a period.

There is **hope** for relieving your period pain.

This usually involves finding a health practitioner who is willing to investigate the *root cause* of the pain, and work with you to make a plan to address that underlying cause that can include diet and lifestyle strategies to improve hormone balance.

Masking the symptoms (eg: using the oral contraceptive pill), rather than treating the root cause will only provide temporary relief. Ask your health practitioner to help you investigate and understand the root cause of the pain and how to treat it.

PERIOD PAIN

During a period, the innermost layer of the uterus (endometrium) is shedding. This means that some discomfort may be felt. Unfortunately, women often experience more than slight discomfort.

Common reasons for period pain:
- Increased prostaglandin production that causes contractions of the uterus in order for blood to be expelled from the body. Too many of a certain kind of prostaglandin can cause excess inflammation
- More sensitive pain fibres in uterus during period
- Period pain may be exaggerated by hormone imbalance, stress, poor overall health, poor gut health, poor diet or lifestyle, and reproductive health conditions.

In some cases, excess period pain can be caused by:
- Conditions such as PCOS, endometriosis, adenomyosis or fibroids
- Ovarian cysts

Severe period pain is a symptom that should be monitored and investigated to find the root cause.

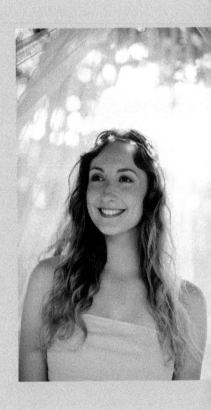

PMS (premenstrual syndrome) is another common period frustration experienced by many women. However, like with period pain, just because it's common, does not mean you have to accept excessive PMS symptoms as normal, especially if they interfere with your ability to carry out everyday life.

WHEN AND WHY DOES PMS HAPPEN?

PMS symptoms can be physical, emotional and behavioural.
These symptoms are noticed during the 'after ovulation' (cat) phase of the menstrual cycle, which lasts for 2 weeks on average, but most women notice the majority of symptoms in the few days before menstruation.
PMS symptoms may arise due to a distinct change in hormones that happens after ovulation. The hormone chart from page 57 shows that after ovulation, **progesterone** levels increase significantly and **oestrogen** levels decrease slightly. This does not mean that progesterone is responsible for your mood swings, sore breasts or fights with your friends. Excessive PMS symptoms may arise when there is an imbalance between these two hormones. There can be a number of underlying causes for this (stress, nutrient deficiency, increased oestrogen exposure, etc.) and symptoms can even be exaggerated by things like sickness, poor diet, lack of exercise, worry or anxiety, and stress due to social factors, school or work. It is important to find a health practitioner who will help you address the root cause.

PMS (Premenstrual syndrome)

Common reasons for PMS:
- A combination of physical, emotional and social influences
- A shift in hormones that takes place in the 2 weeks leading up to a period bleed
- Hormone imbalances, like relative oestrogen excess, can exaggerate symptoms
- Symptoms may also be exaggerated by poor diet and lifestyle habits, and stress

PMS symptoms may include:
- Emotional/mental symptoms
   Eg: Tearfulness, feelings of depression, etc.
- Behavioural symptoms
   Eg: Social withdrawal, changed eating behaviours, etc.
- Physical symptoms
   Eg: Back aches, breast tenderness, acne, headaches, etc.

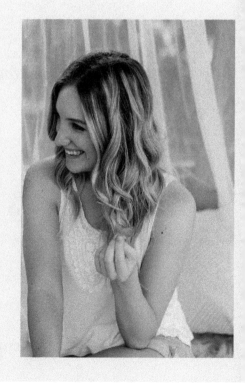

Stress and hormone balance

Prolonged stress can be an enemy to a healthy period, as stress hormones (cortisol and adrenaline) essentially 'fight' with your period hormones (oestrogen and progesterone) and usually win.

When the body is stressed it activates the sympathetic nervous system and initiates what is commonly known as the **fight or flight** response. This is your body's emergency response to danger and is designed to keep you safe. This fight or flight response protects us in a life threatening situation (eg: being chased by a tiger), but also gets activated in non-life threatening situations (eg: public speaking).

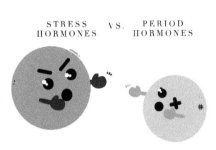

STRESS   VS.   PERIOD
HORMONES   HORMONES

THE BODY'S STRESS RESPONSE

When the fight or flight response is activated, the body's sympathetic nervous system acts to keep us safe from harm. Amongst other things, it works to pump more blood around the body to skeletal muscles, makes breathing more rapid, and increases heart rate and blood sugar. These physical responses require energy and are prioritised in times of stress.

Creating balanced period hormones isn't on the top of our body's priority list if it thinks it's in danger. Therefore, in stressful times we may notice more unwanted period symptoms than usual.

Effects of stress on the menstrual cycle

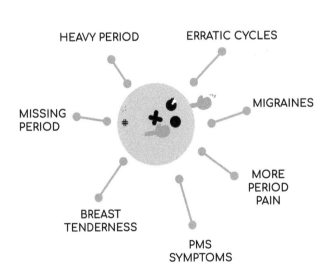

HEAVY PERIOD

ERRATIC CYCLES

MISSING PERIOD

MIGRAINES

MORE PERIOD PAIN

BREAST TENDERNESS

PMS SYMPTOMS

More fight or flight responses:

- Sweating
- Tense muscles
- Tight chest
- Cool or pale skin
- Faster or heavier breathing
- Harder to breathe
- Feeling hot
- Rising blood sugar
- Digestive issues
- Sleep disturbance
- Headaches
- Anxiety

Managing stress

When you recognise you're stressed, it's important to manage that stress and support the body to deactivate the fight or flight response as soon as possible, so it can get back to creating healthy, balanced period hormones. When you notice the signs of stress, use the BEDD acronym to help manage your worries.

B E AWARE of your stressors
Knowing what is making you stressed sounds simple, however, many people will *feel* stressed, but do not identify the cause. When you notice the signs of stress, reflect on the things in your life that may be causing you to feel that way. A friend, mentor or counselor may be able to help.

E LIMINATE the stressors within your control
There are always things you have influence over in a situation, like rescheduling events to give you more time, or even adopting an attitude of thankfulness and positivity within the situation. Focusing on what you're grateful for can crowd out anxious thoughts.

D EVELOP STRATEGIES for what you can't eliminate
Not everything is within your control to change, for example, you can't control the workload you get assigned at school or work. When the cause of stress is not within your control to change, you can decide to adopt a positive attitude and find strategies for handling the stress, like finding a friend or mentor to talk with or help you complete work tasks.

D E-STRESSING techniques incorporated into your daily routine
Do more of what makes you happy, exercise, listen to music, hang out with friends, rest, sleep, colour or draw, play with animals, or incorporate breathing exercise into your day.

Deep breathing exercises for managing stress

1. Breathe in through nose (belly expands) - **4 seconds**

2. Hold breath - **4 second**

3. Breathe out through mouth (belly deflates) - **6 seconds**

Deep breathing can signal to the brain that it is no longer in danger and it can deactivate the fight or flight response.

It can be helpful to stop and breathe consciously when you identify that you're feeling stressed.

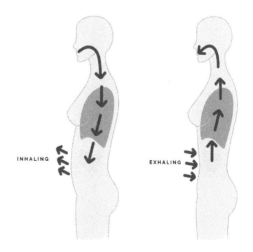

INHALING   EXHALING

The typical period

It is important to remember that everybody's body is different! Not everyone's menstrual cycle will look identical, and that is OK! However, it isn't a good sign for someone's period to look *drastically* different to what is typical. That could be the body's way of communicating an issue that needs investigating.

THE TYPICAL PERIOD

S	M	T	W	T	F	S
	1	2	3	4	5	6
7	8	9	10	11	12	14
15	16	17	18	19	20	21
22	23	24	25	26	27	**28**
29	30	31	32	33	34	35

PERIOD COMES EVERY 21-35 DAYS

The average is 28 days. For adolescents, the typical range is often larger (eg: 20-45 days).

NO EXCESSIVE PAIN

Even if your mum, sister, friends and the girls on social media experience period pain, that doesn't make it normal or good. If pain makes it hard to complete everyday tasks, it should be investigated.

S	M	T	W	T	F	S
1 ♥	2 ♥	3 ♥	4 ♥	5 ♥	6 ♥	7 ♥
8	9	10	11	12	13	14
15	16	17	18	19	20	21
22	23	24	25	26	27	28

BLEEDING LASTS 4-7 DAYS

BLOOD SHOULD BE A RICH, BRIGHT RED COLOUR

Dark brown or watery pink blood is not typical. Some brownish blood at the beginning or end of a period is normal.

NO CLOTS

The typical period has no (or very minimal) clots.

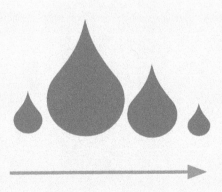

BLOOD FLOW IS LIGHT > HEAVY > LIGHT

Blood flow starts light, becomes heavier for the first few days of bleeding, and becomes lighter again after day 3 or 4. It shouldn't get heavier towards day 6 or 7.

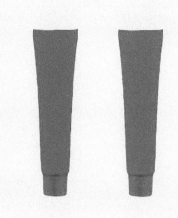

2-4 TABLESPOONS OF BLOOD LOSS...

The average amount of blood loss on a period approximately fills 1-2 tubes of paw paw ointment.

80mL of blood loss is considered a heavy period.

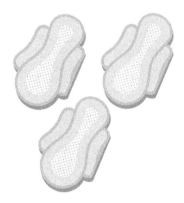

...WHICH IS ROUGHLY

- 3-4 pads/tampons per day
  OR
- 1 pad/tampon every 3-4 hours

Heavy periods may be indicated by needing to change a pad/tampon every 1-2 hours.

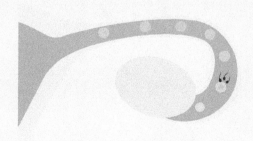

OVULATION ALWAYS HAPPENS

In order for a true period to happen, ovulation needs to occur. It is possible to have a cycle in which ovulation doesn't take place (anovulatory cycle), but this is not typical.

Is it a true period?

Have you ever had 2 periods within 2 weeks? Have you experienced a period that was extremely overdue, and when it finally arrived it looked different and was heavier or lighter than usual? These unusual bleeds may not be true periods.

WHAT CLASSIFIES AS A TRUE PERIOD?

In order for true menstruation to occur, ovulation must happen. Ovulation is an essential part of the menstrual cycle. It is the event that signals a rise in progesterone, a drop in oestrogen and the initiation of the luteal phase (the after ovulation/cat phase) of the menstrual cycle.

It's important to maintain regular cycles in which both ovulation and menstruation occur. This allows for the cyclical release of hormones in the ideal amounts, and prevents them from becoming imbalanced. If ovulation does not occur, the body does not produce progesterone in the required amounts. As progesterone balances out the effects of oestrogen, the absence of ovulation can lead to a range of oestrogen driven complications and symptoms.

ABNORMAL BLEEDS DUE TO ANOVULATION

Anovulation is when ovulation does not happen within a cycle. This can lead to a missing or significantly delayed period. In other cases, a bleed may still occur in an anovulatory cycle and is referred to as an anovulatory bleed. This is not true menstruation. Anovulation is more common in women with PCOS, a thyroid or adrenal condition, or women approaching menopause. Teenagers may experience irregular ovulation in the first few years of menstruation. This usually becomes more regular with time, but should be monitored.

A bleed on the oral contraceptive pill (OCP), is another example of an anovulatory bleed. The purpose of the OCP (and other hormonal contraceptive options) is to stop the body from ovulating. If a woman is not ovulating while on contraception, her body does not go through a menstrual cycle. A bleed on the OCP is a type of anovulatory bleed commonly called a 'withdrawal bleed', as it is a result of a sudden withdrawal from hormone pills when the 7 non-hormone pills are taken.

CHECKLIST TO DETERMINE A TRUE PERIOD

 You've observed a basal body temperature shift that suggests ovulation

 You've observed cervical fluid patterns to reinforce basal body temperature in suggesting ovulation

 You've confirmed ovulation using another method (ovulation kits, doctor visit, etc.)

ABNORMAL BLEEDING

Abnormal bleeding (including anovulatory bleeding) refers to vaginal bleeds that are not a menstrual period. These occur erratically or with unpredictable timing. An abnormal bleed may also differ from the typical period in terms of the colour, quality and flow of the blood, and length of time the bleeding lasts.

Abnormal bleeding should not be ignored. If someone experiences bleeding that is not a true period, has no apparent cause, is painful, and is persistent, it should be brought up with a health practitioner immediately.

OTHER REASONS FOR IRREGULAR BLEEDING

Irregular bleeds may occur for a range of reasons. Considering the large scope of potential causes, it's important to consult with a trusted health practitioner if you experience bleeding that is not part of a regular menstrual cycle.

Potential causes for abnormal bleeding include:
- Pregnancy or miscarriage
- Ovulation spotting
- Vaginal infections
- Endometriosis or adenomyosis
- Use of hormonal contraceptives (speak to a professional if your contraceptive causes persistent abnormal bleeding)
- In some cases, abnormal bleeding can be a sign of cancer of the ovaries, cervix, uterus or endometrium.

There are more causes for abnormal bleeding, ranging from serious to easily treated. Therefore, it's important to work with a professional for an individual diagnosis.

WHEN TO INVESTIGATE ABNORMAL BLEEDING:

Speak with a health practitioner if you observe:

- Bleeding that is continuous and does not stop, or only stops for a short period of time

- Bleeding that happens between a normal menstrual period.
  Ovulation spotting is experienced by some women mid-cycle at ovulation time, and may be observed as 1-2 days of light spotting of brown or pink blood. This is not necessarily a major concern but is not ideal. If it's a regular occurance, see a health practitioner to address the cause

- Unexpected, irregular or persistent bleeds while using contraception

- Bleeds that persistently occur less than 20 days, or more than 36 days apart

- Bleeding that does not reflect the characteristics of a typical period outlined earlier in this chapter

- Bleeding during or after sex

- Any pain associated with abnormal bleeding

Getting to the bottom of period concerns

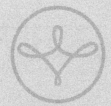

Overcoming period irregularities

Overcoming your period problems is possible, whether you're a teenager or you've been having a period for 20 years.
Periods can be symptom free!
With the right help and guidance from a trusted professional, you can balance your hormones and have a better period.

There is always something you can do to improve your health.

WHAT IS ACCEPTABLE?

Often, women brush off their period irregularities as 'just the way it is', or as something that is 'normal'. Pain and misery shouldn't have to be your normal experience each month. PMS symptoms shouldn't cause you to fight with your friends. Period pain shouldn't mean you physically can't get out of bed.
Periods do not have to be a week of misery.
Let's rethink what we should accept as normal.

ACHIEVABLE HEALTHY PERIOD

- Regular and predictable periods
- Minimal PMS symptoms
- Minimal to no period pain
- Typical blood loss of 2-4 tablespoons
- Bright red blood flow
- Minimal to no clotting
- Regular ovulation
- Stable moods
- Stable eating behaviours
- High energy
- Bleeding for 4-7 days
- Period comes every 21-35 days
- Minimal acne breakouts
- Ability to participate in all activities during period bleed

IRREGULARITIES YOU DON'T NEED TO ACCEPT AS 'NORMAL'

- Extreme PMS
- Bad pain/cramps
- Unpredictable cycles
- Cycles <21 days or >35 days
- Heavy or very light bleeding
- Heavy clotting
- Painful back, breasts, thighs
- Headaches and migraines
- Spotting/bleeding between periods
- Pain between periods
- Anxiety and depression
- Extreme mood swings
- No ovulation (anovulatory cycles)
- Low energy
- Bleeding for <4 or >7 days
- Persistent hormonal acne

Knowing when to seek help

SEEKING HELP FROM PROFESSIONALS

Some girls can be hesitant to see a doctor because they feel embarrassed, scared, or they would prefer not to know if there is an underlying issue.

Most women experience period irregularities in their life. *You're not alone.*

Experiencing a period irregularity doesn't mean something is terribly wrong. It should, however, prompt you to question what might be causing the irregularity.

A lot of period irregularities could have simple solutions that can make a world of difference.

If there is an underlying issue/cause, it's better to catch it sooner than later.

HOW DO I KNOW WHEN TO SEEK HELP FROM A PROFESSIONAL?

1. **Just because it's 'common' doesn't mean it's normal**

Just because you know people who experience a particular period irregularity, that doesn't mean it's 'normal' or 'good' if it is bothering you (ie. horrible period pain, acne, bad mood swings, poor digestion, etc.).

Surveys report that 80% of women experience period pain, varying from mild pain to disabling pain. Just because it's common, doesn't mean you should endure being miserable each month. If this is you, seek solutions!

2. **If a symptom stops you from living your best life, participating in everyday activities and doing the things you want to do**

20-40% of women said that their PMS symptoms were troubling enough to negatively impact their daily life. If period irregularities are stopping you from participating in or carrying out everyday activities, listen to your body and investigate your symptoms further.

3. **Look for patterns**

Something that happens once and never happens again may not be cause to run to the doctor in a worry, unless it's a new or concerning symptom, or the first 2 rules apply. However, when period irregularities form a pattern of arising again and again, it is important to investigate the signs your body is giving you. If you notice recurring period symptoms or irregularities, it can be helpful to:

- *Chart your symptoms* so you can keep track of patterns. Don't just rely on memory. You can also show this chart to a health professional, and they can use it to help get to the bottom of any issues.
- *Look for patterns on your chart* - Do concerning symptoms happen more than once, or do they occur in a particular phase of your cycle?
- *Share with someone* - Telling a parent, friend or partner can help you determine if your symptoms are something other people experience. Your family and friends can also help you look out for patterns.

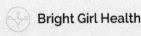 **YouTube**   **BRIGHT GIRL HEALTH** "PCOS and endometriosis story"   🔍

Options for seeking help

Have you ever visited a health professional and been asked you about your period even though it had nothing to do with why you were there?

Doctors ask about periods all the time because period signs and symptoms are our body's intelligent way of communicating things about our health.

Finding a health professional that you trust is important. You deserve to have the best period possible. A health professional can support you to achieve this through tailored guidance to help get you the right treatment and get your health and hormones back on track faster. This might include diet and lifestyle strategies, and even hormone testing.

WHERE TO SEEK HEALTH INFORMATION/ADVICE

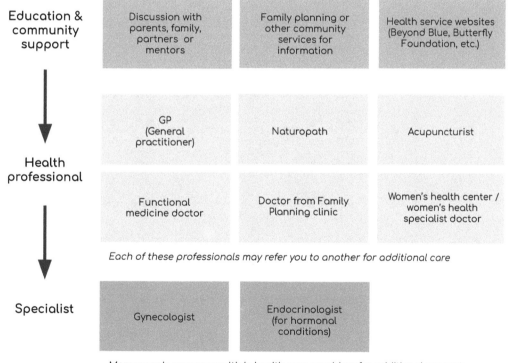

Education & community support

- Discussion with parents, family, partners or mentors
- Family planning or other community services for information
- Health service websites (Beyond Blue, Butterfly Foundation, etc.)

Health professional

- GP (General practitioner)
- Naturopath
- Acupuncturist
- Functional medicine doctor
- Doctor from Family Planning clinic
- Women's health center / women's health specialist doctor

Each of these professionals may refer you to another for additional care

Specialist

- Gynecologist
- Endocrinologist (for hormonal conditions)

Many people may see multiple health care providers for additional support, second opinions or to find the right fit for them. Don't be afraid to try different doctors until you find one that you feel is the right fit for you.

 YouTube   **BRIGHT GIRL HEALTH** "Getting answers about your period from your doctor"   🔍

Options for seeking help

PRACTITIONER	WHAT THEY DO
GP (General practitioner)	This is usually the first place most women go to seek help with period concerns. The costs could be covered by public health care. GPs will be able to order testing and advise you on any other area of your health you may have concerns or questions about. Women's health or reproductive health is not always the specialist area of many GPs, but they can refer you to a specialist who may be able give you further help or advice.
Functional medicine doctor	A functional GP or functional medicine doctor may take a holistic approach to finding the cause of your symptoms, taking into account your history, lifestyle and other aspects of your health.
Women's health centre or GP specialising in women's health	Not all doctors specialise in women's health, but you can find someone who does. A google search for a doctor who specialises in women's health can help you to find doctors in your area. You can also search for a women's health centre, where you can see nurses and doctors who are dedicated to addressing women's health concerns.
Gynecologist	You can ask for a referral to a gynecologist from your GP. Gynecologists are not just for pregnant women! They are specialists in women's health and may be a preferred route for women with hormone disorders, fertility issues, reproductive health conditions, STIs, or specific reproductive health concerns.
Naturopath	Naturopaths are professionals who work to treat the root causes of symptoms through diet, lifestyle, and herbal supplementation. They can recommend more natural approaches to treating and preventing symptoms. Visiting a naturopath for period issues can be beneficial, especially during teenage years when natural treatments, as opposed to pharmaceutical drugs, may be appropriate while your hormones are still regulating.
Acupuncture	Many women find acupuncture helpful to relieve period symptoms and support their hormones. Research shows it helps to reduce inflammation, which can help with common period complaints.
Family Planning services	Family Planning is a not for profit organisation in Australia. They offer a range of health information online for further learning on sexual and reproductive health, as well as a helpline phone number. They also have clinics where appointments can be made to see a doctor. If you're located outside Australia, search for similar sexual health organisations in your area.

TRUST YOUR GUT!

If you don't think that the kind of symptoms you experience are normal, look into it, do research, ask questions & talk to a professional.
If you're not happy with an experience you have with a particular practitioner,
seek a second opinion!

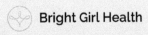 Bright Girl Health

Appreciate your body

If you take away one thing from reading this book, remember that your body and your period are amazing and intelligent. Each day your body works to keep you healthy and safe without you having to consciously think about it! The period symptoms you experience are your body's way of communicating to you.

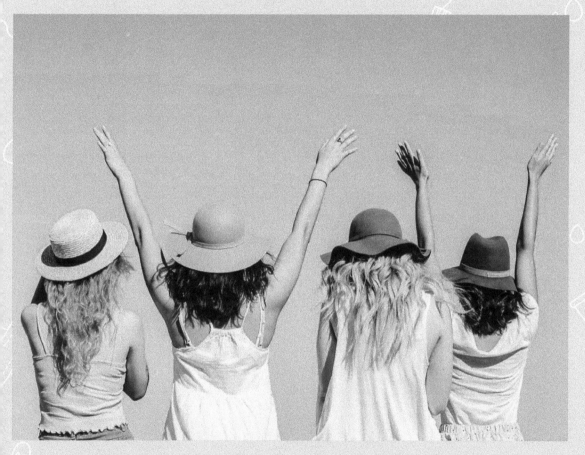

Remember that your body and your period can speak... and you can choose to listen.

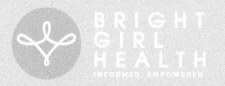

MY DOCTOR SAYS I'M FINE BUT I DON'T FEEL FINE. WHAT DO I DO?

If this is how you feel, you're not alone.
Here are some suggestions:

1. **TRUST YOUR GUT**
   If the period symptoms you experience are impacting your everyday life and you've thought "this just can't be normal", keep persisting in your search for answers.

2. **TRACK ANY PATTERNS**
   Track ALL your period symptoms on an app or paper chart. Write down EVERYTHING. Look for patterns that may arise. You can show this to your doctor to help them understand the weight and nature of your concerns.

3. **ASK FOR A HORMONE TEST**
   If you feel you've tried everything but your period is still giving you trouble, ask your doctor for a hormone test. This may help uncover part of the cause of your symptoms. However, your doctor will need a *reason* to have your hormones tested, because testing costs money, and they may not order tests without a clear reason. Showing a doctor your recorded symptoms can help to demonstrate enough cause to have these tests done.

4. **SEEK A SECOND OPINION**
   If you feel as though you haven't got the answers that explain your period symptoms, there is nothing wrong with seeking a second opinion (or third or fourth!) from a different doctor. You may also ask your doctor for a referral to a women's health specialist for more specific help. Finding a health professional that is a good fit for you may take a while, but is worth it.

CAN A TAMPON OR MENSTRUAL CUP GET LOST INSIDE MY VAGINA?

Tampons and menstrual cups sit inside the vaginal canal, but below your cervix.
The cervix is like the 'gateway' into your uterus. The opening of the cervix is only about the size of a pen tip. It is not possible for a tampon or menstrual cup to move past the cervix, considering this opening is so small.
No matter how high within the vaginal canal the tampon or menstrual cup sits, it will stay within the canal.

If you find your menstrual cup has moved higher, bearing down, squatting and reaching for it with 2 fingers should put it within reach. It is also important to relax, as tensing can move it further out of reach.

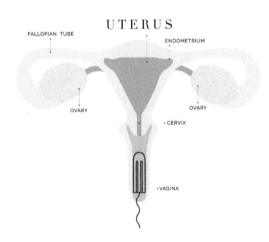

UTERUS

FALLOPIAN TUBE

ENDOMETRIUM

OVARY

OVARY

CERVIX

VAGINA

FAQs

I'M 16 AND HAVEN'T HAD MY FIRST PERIOD. SHOULD I BE WORRIED?

Lots of girl experience their first period after the age of 16. This is referred to as primary amenorrhea. Sometimes it can be frustrating when your body doesn't do what you would like it to.

A missing period can be your body's way of talking to you, telling you there is something that it needs or something that it's lacking. A missing period is missing for a reason. There can be a range of reasons - but it doesn't necessarily need to be a cause for panic!

Some things that can contribute to a girl getting her first period later include existing health conditions, eating disorders, excessive exercise or serious athleticism, genetics, etc.

Chatting with a trusted medical professional if your period hasn't shown up is a great idea to stay on top of your health and ensure that other areas of your health aren't hindering you from getting your first period.

WHY DOES PERIOD BLOOD TURN BROWN?

Period blood can start to turn brown when exposed to oxygen. Sometimes period blood is brownish at the very beginning or end of the bleed. This can be because the blood flow is lighter on the first and last day of a period, meaning it moves out of the body more slowly and is exposed to oxygen for longer.

WHY DOES PERIOD BLOOD SMELL?

Period blood can start to smell when it is exposed to oxygen.
This can be why using a pad, and even a tampon, can become a bit smelly after a few hours.

MY PERIOD IS MISSING. SHOULD I BE WORRIED?

The first thing you should ask yourself is, "is this a pattern?".
In other words, does it keep happening?
If your period goes missing for 3 weeks while you're going through a big life change or stressful situation but comes back and returns to normal like nothing ever happened - then that may not be a cause for concern (unless you experience additional unwanted or concerning symptoms).

However, if your period has a pattern or habit of going missing, then it can be empowering to get to the root cause. Usually a period will go missing because ovulation is not happening. Ovulation can be hindered by many things - stress, nutrient deficiency, coming off the pill, poor overall health, medical issues, eating disorders, extreme exercise, etc. It's really important that you get to the cause of WHY you're not ovulating after speaking with a medical professional and even getting some hormone tests done.

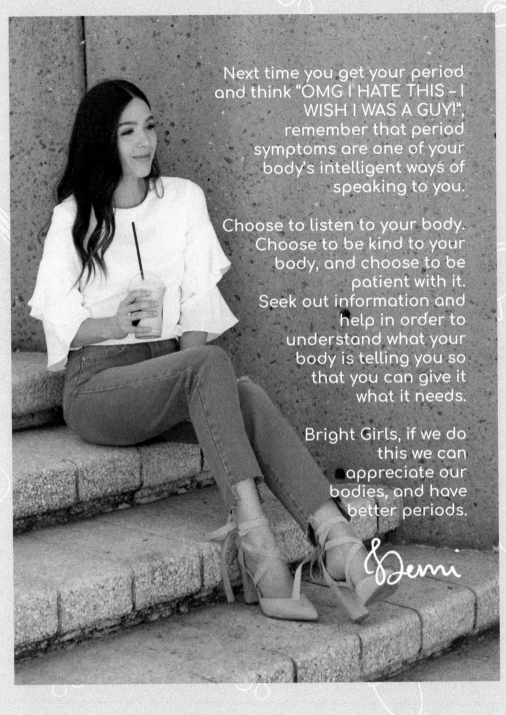

Next time you get your period and think "OMG I HATE THIS – I WISH I WAS A GUY!", remember that period symptoms are one of your body's intelligent ways of speaking to you.

Choose to listen to your body. Choose to be kind to your body, and choose to be patient with it. Seek out information and help in order to understand what your body is telling you so that you can give it what it needs.

Bright Girls, if we do this we can appreciate our bodies, and have better periods.

Demi

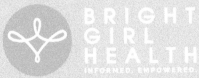

BRIGHT
GIRL
HEALTH
INFORMED. EMPOWERED.

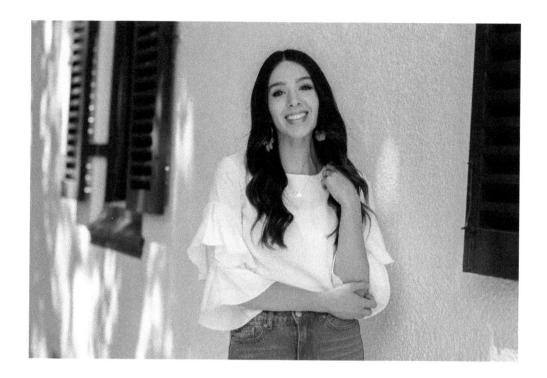

ABOUT DEMI

Demi is the founder of Bright Girl Health, a women's health educator and a passionate high school teacher. She believes that girls should never feel left in the dark about their own body.
Demi loves banana smoothie bowls, binge watching Netflix, hanging out with her hubby, and she can kind of do a handstand.

"Growing up, I knew next to nothing about my period and my body. I realised that a lot of guys actually knew more about periods than I did!
When I was in my early twenties I decided to learn more about how my period works by reading 'Taking Charge of Your Fertility' and couldn't put the book down because every page was blowing my mind with new information I didn't know about my own body!
After realising how my body worked I had a new appreciation for my period and felt **empowered** *to use it to my advantage! I wanted to write this book so that others, especially young women, can experience the same feeling of empowerment as I did."*

Understanding reproductive health is an obstacle many young girls face because of embarrassment, shame, lack of resources, shying away from 'taboos', and misinformation from the media or friends. Demi's goal is to break through the silence when it comes to discussing women's health.

DISCLAIMER

The use of any information or recommendations in this book is at your own risk. It is the individual's responsibility, alongside a medical professional, to ensure that any health services, recommendations or information you act upon meet your specific requirements.
You are responsible for seeking advice from your a healthcare professional before acting on any information in this book.
Any health concerns, pre-existing medical conditions or questions regarding your health should be brought up with your doctor.

The information and advice given in this book is not provided as medical or
professional advice or opinion. The information given in this book does not take into account individual circumstances or health history.

Demi Spaccavento hereby avoids liability and/or responsibility for any adverse outcomes that might arise, directly or indirectly, from any recommendations in this book.

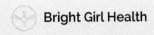

REFERENCES

Akgül S., Başaran H.O., Cetin M., Derman O., Gümrük F., & Kanbur N.O. (2013). Dysfunctional uterine bleeding in adolescent girls and evaluation of their response to treatment. *The Turkish Journal of Pediatrics. 55(2)*, 186-189. Retrieved from https://www.ncbi.nlm.nih.gov/pubmed/24192679

Baker, C., Waner, J., Vieira, E., Taylor, S., Driver, H., & Mitchell, D. (2004). Sleep and 24 hour body temperatures: a comparison in young men, naturally cycling women and women taking hormonal contraceptives. *The Journal of Physiology, 530*(3), 565–574. doi: http://doi.org/10.1111/j.1469-7793.2001.0565k.x

Bigelow, J., Dunson, DB., Stanford, JB., Ecochard, R., Gnoth, C., & Colombo, B. (2004). Mucus observations in the fertile window: a better predictor of conception than timing of intercourse. *Human Reproduction. 19*(4), 889-892. doi: 10.1093/humrep/deh173.

BodyTalk. (2018a). Girl Stuff. *Family Planning NSW.* Retrieved from https://bodytalk.org.au/puberty/girl-stuff/

BodyTalk. (2018b). How Pregnancy Happens. *Family Planning NSW.* Retrieved from https://bodytalk.org.au/how-it-works/conception-how-pregnancy-happens/

BodyTalk. (2018c). Menstruation. *Family Planning NSW.* Retrieved from https://bodytalk.org.au/how-it-works/menstruation/

Bradley, L. D. (2004). Vaginal Bleeding. In S. Loue, & M. Sajatovic (Eds.), *Encyclopedia of women's health*. Dordrecht, The Netherlands: Springer Science+Business Media. Retrieved from http://databases.avondale.edu.au/login?url=https://search.credoreference.com/content/entry/sprwh/vaginal_bleeding/0?institutionId=6415

Jardim, N. (2014). *Get to Know the 4 Phases of your Menstrual Cycle.* Retrieved from https://www.mindbodygreen.com/0-16167/get-to-know-the-4-phases-of-your-menstrual-cycle.html

Knight, J. (2017). *The Complete Guide to Fertility Awareness* (1st ed.). New York: Routledge.

Kringoudis, N. (2014). *Well and Good.* Melbourne: Melbourne University Press.

Mansfield, M.J., & Emans, S,J. (1984). Adolescent menstrual irregularity. *Journal of Reproductive Medicine. 29*(6), 399-410.

Menstrual Cycle. (2012). In R. Sell, M. A. Rothenberg, & C. F. Chapman, *Dictionary of Medical Terms* (6th ed.). Hauppauge, NY: Barron's Educational Series. Retrieved from http://databases.avondale.edu.au/login?url=https://search.credoreference.com/content/entry/barronsm/menstrual_cycle/0?institutionId=6415

Marzieh, R. D., Fahimeh, R. T., Djalalinia, S., Cheraghi, L., Samira, B. G., & Azizi, F. (2016). Menstrual cycle irregularity and metabolic disorders: A population-based prospective study. *PLoS One, 11*(12). doi:http://dx.doi.org.databases.avondale.edu.au/10.1371/journal.pone.0168402

Mayo, J. L. (1997). A healthy menstrual cycle. *Clin Nutr Insights, 5*(9), 1-8.∠

OpenStax. (2013). *Anatomy and Physiology.* Houston, TX: OpenStax CNX. Retrieved from https://opentextbc.ca/anatomyandphysiology

Owen, M. (2013). Physiological signs of ovulation and fertility readily observable by women. *The Linacre Quarterly. 80*(1), 17-23. Retrieved from https://www.ncbi.nlm.nih.gov/pubmed/24845657

Popat, V. B., Prodanov, T., Calis, K. A., & Nelson, L. M. (2008). The Menstrual Cycle A Biological Marker of General Health in Adolescents. *Annals of the New York Academy of Sciences, 1135*, 43–51. http://doi.org/10.1196/annals.1429.040

Pope, A. (2010). Follow Your Natural Cycle. *Psychologies.* Retrieved from http://janebennett.com.au/admin/wp-content/uploads/2011/03/1Natural-Cycle-Psychologies-Sept-2010.pdf

Reed B. G., & Carr B. R. (2000). The Normal Menstrual Cycle and the Control of Ovulation. In *Endotext - 22 May, 2015*. South Dartmouth, Massachusetts: MDText.com, Inc. Retrieved from https://www.ncbi.nlm.nih.gov/books/NBK279054/

Rao, K.A. (2009). *Textbook of Gynaecology* (1st ed.). India: Elsevier.

The Royal Women's Hospital Victoria Australia. (2018). *Ovulation and conception.* Retrieved from https://www.thewomens.org.au/health-information/fertility-information/getting-pregnant/ovulation-and-conception

Trickey, R. (2011). *Women, Hormones and the Menstrual cycle* (3rd ed.). Victoria, Australia: Trickey Enterprises.

Weschler, T. (2015). *Taking Charge of Your Fertility: The Definitive Guide to Natural Birth Control, Pregnancy Achievement, and Reproductive Health* (20th Anniversary edition). Harper Collins.

Wilcox, A. J., Dunson, D., & Baird, D. D. (2000). The timing of the "fertile window" in the menstrual cycle: day specific estimates from a prospective study. *British Medical Journal, 321*(7271), 1259–1262.

World Health Organisation. (1988). *Natural Family Planning: A guide to provision of services.* Retrieved from http://apps.who.int/iris/bitstream/handle/10665/39322/9241542411-eng.pdf?sequence=1&isAllowed=y

CPSIA information can be obtained
at www.ICGtesting.com
Printed in the USA
BVHW092110130822
644541BV00003B/3